VASCULAR ANATOMY AND PHYSIOLOGY

AN INTRODUCTORY TEXT

VASCULAR ANATOMY AND PHYSIOLOGY

AN INTRODUCTORY TEXT

ANN C. BELANGER, RN, RVT

Foreword by
Victor M. Bernhard, MD

DAVIES
Registry Reviews & Study Aids

SDMS-Approved
Continuing Education Activity
Approved for 5 hours CME Credit

DAVIES PUBLISHING

Library of Congress Cataloging-in-Publication Data

Belanger, Ann C., 1947 –
Vascular anatomy and physiology: an introductory text / Ann C. Belanger; foreword by Victor M. Bernhard.
p. cm.
Includes bibliographical references.
Includes index.
ISBN 0-941022-11-0
1. Blood-vessels—Physiology. 2. Blood-vessels—Anatomy.
I. Title.
[DNLM: 1. Blood Circulation—physiology. 2. Blood Vessels— anatomy & histology. WG 101 B426v]
QP106.B44 1990
612. 1'3—dc20
DNLM/DLC
for Library of Congress

90-925
CIP

Davies Publishing Inc.
32 South Raymond Avenue
Pasadena, California 91105-1935
Phone: (626) 792-3046
Fax: (626) 792-5308
Website: DaviesPublishing.com

Illustrations by Stephen Beebe.
Copy editing and electronic manuscript by Lillian R. Rodberg & Associates.
Cover and text design by Graphics Two.

Printed and bound in the United States of America.

ISBN 978-0-941022-11-8

This book is lovingly dedicated to my parents, Catherine and Harvey, whose love, support, and encouragement have been constant throughout my life.

Foreword

This basic and well-written primer will be a true asset to the education of vascular and radiology technologists, sonographers, nurses, and others who seek a clear and simple presentation of the pertinent facts about vascular anatomy and physiology. Indeed, the author has done an admirable job of providing basic information in a clear and succinct fashion. Her choice of language to describe problems encountered by vascular technologists is readily understandable and therefore applicable to people from diverse backgrounds who are seeking technical proficiency in the expanding field of noninvasive technology for the evaluation of vascular diseases.

The author brings to her text a long experience in direct application of vascular testing and also in teaching the fundamentals that are required for proficiency in this field. An excellent basic bibliography is provided for those students who are intellectually more curious. Illustrations are clear and effectively augment the text. This book will be valuable to the advanced trainee preparing for certification, as well as to the beginning student.

Victor M. Bernhard, MD
Professor of Surgery and Chief, Section of Vascular Surgery
University of Arizona Health Sciences Center

Preface

This book is intended to introduce the normal anatomy and physiology of the human vascular system. I hope that it will provide a basis for understanding to those entering the fields of vascular technology, radiologic technology, sonography, nursing and related health care professions. It may also be useful to anyone who simply wants to know how his or her body works. It is not intended to be a comprehensive textbook or a definitive reference on the subject.

The field of noninvasive vascular diagnosis has attracted practitioners from diverse backgrounds. Some have come from other areas of health care—nursing, respiratory therapy, x-ray/ultrasound, and the like. Many others have had no previous health care experience. It is generally easy to teach newcomers the mechanics of testing. But unless they understand the "why" as well as the "how" of testing, they will never become truly proficient. To understand the "why" of testing, a knowledge of vascular pathology is important, and one cannot really understand abnormalities without first having a clear understanding of the normal.

In teaching both the novice and the experienced vascular technologist, it became apparent to me that a comprehensive knowledge of the normal anatomy and physiology of the vascular system was commonly wanting. There are many texts that detail the techniques of performing vascular tests. There are also excellent sources of information on the pathological processes requiring testing. There seemed, however, to be a lack of readily available and understandable information about the *normal* vascular system. Moreover, most of the texts and references that were available presupposed the reader's familiarity with medical terminology. This text, on the other hand, focuses on the normal anatomy and physiology of the vascular system, and it is designed to be easily understood even by those readers with little or no previous medical training.

In order to gain the most from the text, it is strongly advised that you utilize both the pretest and the final examination found at the end of the book. Both tests are written in an objective, multiple-choice format, and each question has only one correct answer. You should take the pretest before reading the text. After completing the text, retake the pretest and compare results. If you find areas in which you still lack confidence—the venous anatomy, for instance—review that section before taking the final exam.

The human body is a fascinating thing. It is the most perfect factory ever designed, with each machine functioning more effectively than anything man has yet to devise. Within this complex and intricate human body, the vascular system plays not only the most crucial role (after all, without blood we wouldn't be alive) but, at least in this author's opinion, the most interesting one.

Acknowledgments

The author deeply appreciates the assistance and support she received from many friends.

I wish to thank the many students whose questions provided the inspiration for this book. I've learned as much from them as they, I hope, have learned from me.

I also especially wish to thank Dr. Victor M. Bernhard, Chief of Vascular Surgery at the University of Arizona Health Sciences Center, for his assistance and support as a resource, guide, and manuscript reviewer.

Additionally, I wish to acknowledge the vascular surgeons of Henry Ford Hospital, Detroit, Michigan, who were my original mentors, teachers, and guides into and through the world of vascular diagnosis. Dr. Roger Smith, Chairman of the Department of Surgery, provided support as I made the transition from vascular intensive care nurse to vascular laboratory nurse. Dr. Joseph Elliott, the Director of the Henry Ford Vascular Laboratory, my constant source of information and strength, made this transition both a pleasant and an intellectually satisfying experience. And, finally, Dr. D. Emerick Szilagyi—one of the foremost vascular surgeons of our time—taught me not only to read angiograms and venograms, but also to appreciate fully all of the intricacies of the human vascular system. Thank you, gentlemen.

Lastly, and most importantly, I wish to thank my partner and my friend, Elizabeth G. Newton, without whose continuous assistance and support this book never would have been written. Bette has provided not only moral support, but valuable assistance in the structure and execution of this text. By periodically reviewing the manuscript-in-progress, she made certain that the text did not stray from the original concepts of clarity and simplicity. It was also she who first encouraged me to accept the challenge of writing this book and who constantly reassured me of its progress. Thank you, Bette.

Contents

Pretest

Before you begin reading *Vascular Anatomy and Physiology,* answer the following questions on a separate sheet of paper and score yourself by referring to the list of correct answers that appears at the end of this test. Then set the test aside. Once you have finished reading this book, retake the pretest to measure your progress and to identify any remaining areas of weakness. The results will indicate not only how much you have learned about vascular anatomy and physiology but also which topics still present problems for you. Be sure to study those topics again. Remember that there is only one best answer to each of these questions.

QUESTIONS

1. Which of the following arteries is a part of the circle of Willis?
   - A. The internal maxillary artery.
   - B. The supraorbital artery.
   - C. The anterior communicating artery.
   - D. The superior mesenteric artery.
   - E. The occipital artery.

2. Which of the following sets of arteries represents a normal pattern of progression (proximal to distal)?
   - A. Subclavian artery to radial artery to brachial artery.
   - B. Abdominal aorta to superior mesenteric artery to inferior mesenteric artery.
   - C. Aortic arch to internal carotid artery to external carotid artery.
   - D. Abdominal aorta to common iliac artery to external iliac artery.
   - E. Common femoral artery to deep femoral artery to superficial femoral artery.

3. The middle layer in the wall of an artery is called:
    A. The tunica intima.
    B. The tunica medicus.
    C. The tunica media.
    D. The tunica middle.
    E. The tunica adventitia.

4. The middle layer in the wall of a vein is called:
    A. The tunica intima.
    B. The tunica medicus.
    C. The tunica media.
    D. The tunica middle.
    E. The tunica adventitia.

5. The right and left common iliac veins anastomose to form which vessel?
    A. The inferior mesenteric vein.
    B. The descending abdominal vena cava.
    C. The inferior vena cava.
    D. The superior vena cava.
    E. The abdominal aortic vein.

6. Which three arteries normally arise directly from the aortic arch?
    A. The internal carotid, external carotid, and common carotid arteries.
    B. The right common carotid, innominate, and left common carotid arteries.
    C. The innominate, brachiocephalic, and left common carotid arteries.
    D. The brachiocephalic, right common carotid, and right subclavian arteries.
    E. The brachiocephalic, left common carotid, and left subclavian arteries.

7. From which area in the heart does the ascending thoracic aorta arise?
    A. The right atrium.
    B. The left atrium.
    C. The right ventricle.
    D. The left ventricle.
    E. The left auricle.

8. What is the landmark for bifurcation of the abdominal aorta?
    A. The inguinal ligament.
    B. The popliteal fossa.
    C. The adductor canal.
    D. The umbilicus.
    E. The iliac crest.

9. What kind of energy is considered the energy of motion?
    A. Kinetic energy.
    B. Potential energy.
    C. Mobile energy.
    D. Gravitational energy.
    E. Hydrostatic energy.

10. What is the landmark for the route of the femoral vein?
    A. The inguinal ligament.
    B. The adductor canal.
    C. The umbilicus.
    D. The lateral malleolus.
    E. The carotid canal.

11. Which of the following is <u>not</u> a deep vein?
    A. The femoral vein.
    B. The subclavian vein.
    C. The cephalic vein.
    D. The posterior tibial vein.
    E. The common femoral vein.

12. All of the following veins are located in the upper extremity. Which is a part of the superficial venous system?
    A. The ulnar vein.
    B. The brachial vein.
    C. The basilic vein.
    D. The axillary vein.
    E. The radial vein.

13. Which of the following terms describes a normal characteristic of arterial blood flow?
    A. Phasicity.
    B. Turbulence.
    C. Transitoriness.
    D. Vacillation.
    E. Pulsatility.

14. Which of the following landmarks is used to locate the normal position of the carotid bifurcation?
    A. The carotid canal.
    B. The clavicle.
    C. The masseter muscle.
    D. The thyroid cartilage.
    E. The inguinal ligament.

15. Which of the following terms is used to describe a normal characteristic of lower-extremity venous blood flow?
    A. Pulsatility.
    B. Steadiness.
    C. Turbulence.
    D. Swiftness.
    E. Phasicity.

ANSWERS

1.	C.	6.	E.	11.	C.
2.	D.	7.	D.	12.	C.
3.	C.	8.	D.	13.	E.
4.	C.	9.	A.	14.	D.
5.	C.	10.	B.	15.	E.

SECTION ONE

Anatomic Terminology

Much of the terminology used in medicine comes from ancient Latin or Greek. Sometimes the words have evolved into modified forms of the original; at other times, the words we use today are exactly the same as those spoken by early Romans and Greeks. An understanding of these terms is important in learning about the structure and function of the human body.

In this book, a great deal of medical terminology is explained in the course of describing the anatomy and physiology of the vascular system. However, before we can begin exploring the veins and arteries, you will need to know some basic anatomic terms. For example, medical professionals use certain basic terms to describe the different divisions within the body and to indicate directions of movement in reference to the body. These terms are used often throughout this text.

CHAPTER

1

Planes, Areas, and Regions

One of the first concepts you need to understand in learning anatomy is that of normal anatomic position. When one looks at an anatomic drawing showing only the blood vessels, there is no face or other external feature to identify whether the front or the back of the body is being viewed. That is where the normal anatomic position comes into use.

NORMAL ANATOMIC POSITION

Unless otherwise identified, all anatomic illustrations are assumed to be drawn or photographed with the body in the *normal anatomic position*: facing the viewer, with the palmar surface of the hands facing outward. The experience somewhat resembles looking at a mirror image: The viewer's right hand is on the same side as the figure's left, and vice-versa. By always keeping that example in mind, you can avoid confusing the right and left sides of anatomic illustrations and will not wonder which side of an arm or leg is being described.

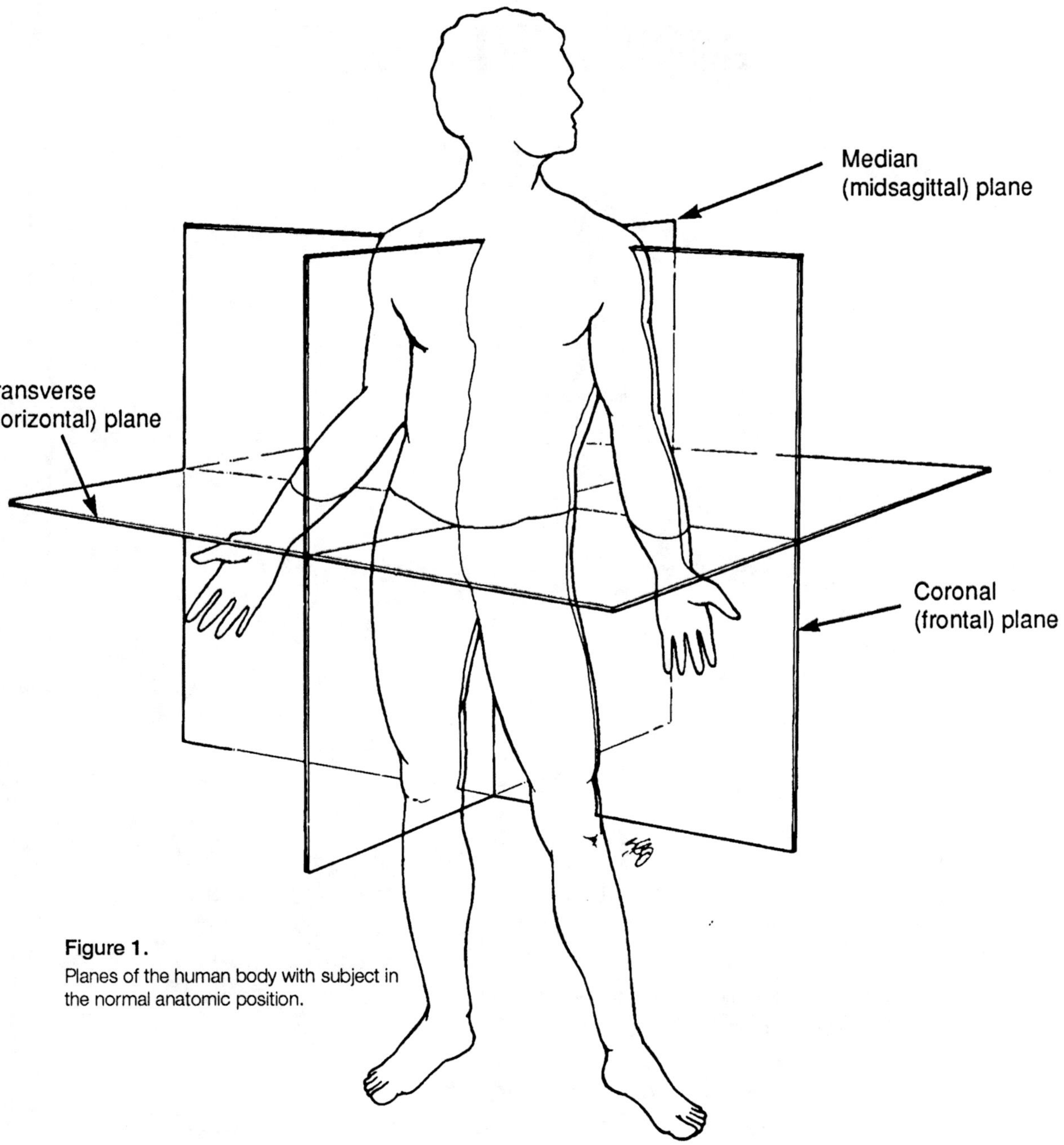

Figure 1.
Planes of the human body with subject in the normal anatomic position.

PLANES OF THE HUMAN BODY

The human body can be mentally divided into many different areas or portions, depending on what is being described. You learned some of these portions as a child. For instance, even a preschooler knows where to find a person's head, arms, or legs. Now you will be learning the more precise ways of defining body areas that are used by medical professionals. One of these methods consists of dividing the body into *planes* by cutting it from top to bottom, from front to back, or through the middle (Figure 1).

First, visualize a body standing before you. Then picture that body being evenly divided between the right and left halves by being cut from the top of the head downward. You have separated the body along its *sagittal plane.* This right/left division may be centered exactly through the midline of the body, or it may be off center. If the division is through the middle, it is called a *median* or *midsagittal* section (*section* in anatomy means a cut or division).

If, instead, the body standing before you is divided into a front and a back half, we are speaking of its *coronal planes* (sometimes called the <u>frontal planes</u>).

Last, the body can be divided the way a magician would "saw a woman in half," that is, across the body, dividing it into top and bottom portions. In anatomy, this is called dividing the body along its *transverse plane*, sometimes called the <u>horizontal plane.</u>

These terms can be applied to parts of the body as well as to the whole. For instance, if you were talking about a thigh, you could discuss its sagittal, coronal, and transverse planes by making imaginary cuts, or sections, in the directions just described. To review:

- The sagittal plane divides the body vertically into right and left sides; if the division is through the midline and creates equal halves, it is called the median, or median sagittal, plane.
- The coronal, or frontal, plane divides the body into front and back halves.
- The transverse, or horizontal, plane cuts across the body, dividing it into upper and lower portions.

In addition to sectioning the body by planes, we can also divide it by body regions, or areas.

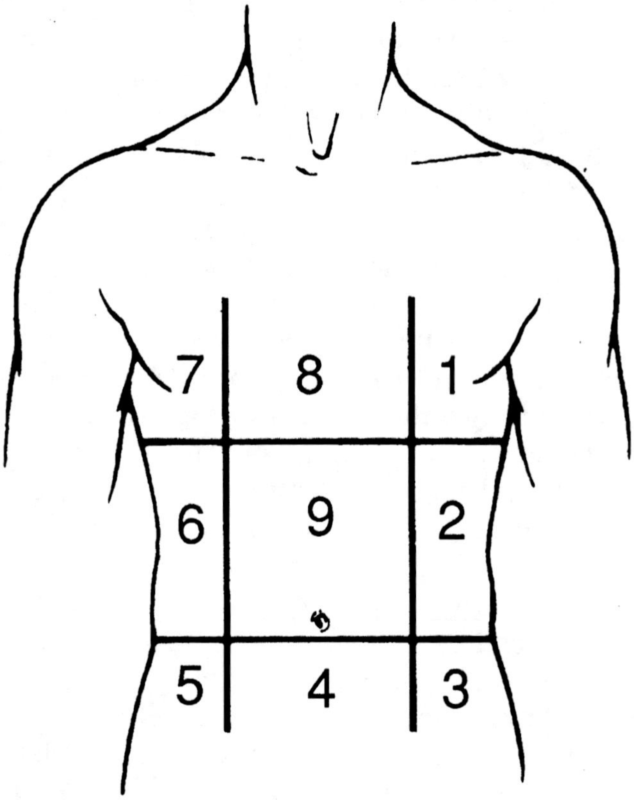

Figure 2.
Regions of the abdomen: 1, left hypochondriac; 2, left lumbar (or lateral); 3, left iliac (or inguinal); 4, hypogastric (or pubic); 5, right iliac (or inguinal); 6, right lumbar (or lateral); 7, right hypochondriac; 8, epigastric; 9, umbilical.

REGIONS OF THE BODY

The three major regions of the body are referred to as the head, or cephalic region; the trunk; and the extremities. The *trunk*, which is the major portion of the body, is formed by the *thorax*, or chest, and the *abdomen*. The *upper extremities* extend outward from the upper portion of each side of the trunk. Although most people refer to the arm as the upper extremity, that is not really correct. The arm, technically, is only that portion of the upper extremity that extends from the shoulder to the elbow. The portion that begins at the elbow and ends at the wrist is called the forearm, with the hand and the digits (fingers) making up the remainder of each upper extremity.

The *lower extremities* are attached to the base of the trunk. These are also subdivided. The attachment of the lower extremity to the trunk is called the inguinal ligament. The area between the thigh and the abdomen is the groin. It is common to refer to the entire lower limb as the leg, but that, too, is incorrect. The upper portion of the lower limb is properly called the thigh and ends at the knee. The section beginning with the knee and ending at the ankle, which is commonly known as the calf, is correctly called the leg. The true calf is the fleshy portion at the back of the leg. The remainder of the lower extremity consists of the foot and the digits (toes).

The body is also referred to in terms of its two major cavities: the chest cavity, known as the *thorax*, or *thoracic cavity*, and the *abdomen*, or *abdominal cavity*.

To make it easier to describe the location of organs, lesions (disease or injury), or pain, the abdominal cavity is commonly subdivided into regions. One subdivision resembles a tic-tac-toe board, with two vertical and two horizontal lines marking off nine separate areas (Figure 2). The upper horizontal line is placed at the level of the ninth rib cartilage; the lower horizontal line is at the level of the iliac crest (the crest of the iliac, or hip, bones). The right and left imaginary vertical lines are drawn upward from the middle of the right and left inguinal ligaments. Beginning with the upper left region and traveling clockwise, we have the:

1. left hypochondriac region
2. left lumbar region
3. left iliac region
4. hypogastric region
5. right iliac region
6. right lumbar region

7. right hypochondriac region
8. epigastric region

and, in the middle:

9. the umbilical region, the region containing the umbilicus, or navel (commonly known as the belly button)

Another way of sectioning the abdomen is in *quadrants*, or quarters. With this method, there is only one vertical and one horizontal line, each passing through the center of the abdomen. Beginning, again, at upper left and proceeding clockwise, these sections are called:

1. the left upper quadrant
2. the left lower quadrant
3. the right lower quadrant
4. the right upper quadrant

CHAPTER REVIEW

- The normal anatomic position always places the figure facing the viewer, with the palmar surface of the hands facing outward.
- The body, and its various parts, can be divided into planes: sagittal; median or midsagittal; coronal or frontal; and transverse or horizontal.
- The three major regions of the body are the head or cephalic region; the trunk; and the extremities.
- The upper extremity consists of the arms (from shoulder to elbow), the forearms (from elbow to wrist), the hands, and the digits (fingers).
- The lower extremity consists of the thighs (from groin to knee), the legs (from knee to ankle), the feet, and the digits (toes).
- The chest cavity is also called the thorax or thoracic cavity; the abdomen is also called the abdominal cavity.
- The abdomen can be divided into either nine or four regions. The nine regions are the left hypochondriac, left lumbar, left iliac, hypogastric, right iliac, right lumbar, right hypochondriac, epigastric, and umbilical. The four regions are the left upper quadrant, left lower quadrant, right lower quadrant, and right upper quadrant.

CHAPTER

2

Direction and Location

Medicine has many terms to describe direction and location. Sometimes they are used to indicate the direction in which something is being or should be moved, for example, "proximally" or "distally." Sometimes, terms give you the direction or location relative to a specific anatomic structure, for example, "infraclavicularly."

TERMS INDICATING DIRECTION

If we wish to indicate that something lies or is moving in the direction of the head, we can use any of three different terms, all meaning the same thing:

- *cranial* or *craniad*
- *superior*
- *cephalad*

All of these words mean that the thing to which you are referring is closer to the "head end" than to the "tail end" of the body, or that it is moving in that direction. For example, the thorax is superior to the abdomen; the neck is cranial to the thorax; or, blood flow in the ascending thoracic aorta moves in a cephalad fashion.

Now, let's say you wish to describe something as being closer to the feet than to the head. The terms you would use in that situation would be:

- *caudal* or *caudad*
- *inferior*

For example, the calf is inferior to the thigh; the abdomen is caudal to the thorax; or, blood flow in the descending thoracic aorta moves in a caudad fashion (or caudally).

The front half of the body is said to be its *anterior* half, or side. Another word for front is *ventral*. So, you could say either that the umbilicus is on the anterior side of the trunk, or that it is on the ventral side. Either would be correct.

To discuss the opposite of the anterior/ventral half, you again have the choice of two words—*posterior* or *dorsal*. If you were describing the nape of the neck, you could choose between saying that the nape is on the posterior aspect of the neck or on the dorsal aspect. (*Aspect* means side.)

Finally, we have words that pertain to movement toward and away from the midline of the body. The term for "toward the midline" is *medial*. The term for "away from the midline" is *lateral*. These terms can be used to compare the locations of different structures or to define the location of one structure. For example, the big toe lies medial to (closer to the midline than) the little toe; the little toe lies lateral to (farther from the midline than) the big toe. Or, using the umbilicus again, we can describe its location as medially in the abdomen. The ear, described as a single structure, lies on the lateral aspect of the head.

In using these directions, you must keep the normal anatomic position in mind. Remember that the imaginary figure has its hands turned so that the palms are facing you. Therefore, the thumb is located on the lateral aspect of the hand, and the "pinkie"

is at the medial side. This is an important point to remember, especially when we begin discussing pulse sites in the upper extremity.

POSITION RELATIVE TO ANOTHER STRUCTURE

Terms that indicate position relative to another structure are often in the form of a directional prefix plus a root that tells us what structure is being described. Commonly used directional prefixes are:

infra- intra- ante- sub- supra- inter- post-

The prefix *infra-* is used to indicate that something is, or should be done, below the thing that is identified by the root. For example, to say that something is infraclavicular is to say that it is located below the clavicle (the collarbone). For instance, you can most easily palpate the subclavian artery by placing your fingers infraclavicularly in the right location. *Supra-* means just the opposite; it means that something is above whatever the root is naming.

People often confuse intra- and inter-. The prefix *intra-* means within; for example, the brain is in the intracranial cavity. *Inter-*, on the other hand, means between. For instance, the wall between the two ventricles of the heart is interventricular.

To indicate that something comes before something else, we can use the prefix *ante-*. So, if something happens before birth, it happens antepartum. Something that occurs after something else is indicated by the prefix *post-*; an after-birth event is called postpartum. Finally, if the direction we wish to indicate is below something, the prefix is *sub-*. The subclavian artery is called that because it lies below the clavicle.

COMBINING DIRECTIONAL TERMS

Directional terms can be combined with other words, including those we defined earlier. Usually, the combining form -o- is used to link two terms. To indicate that something is both in front of and on the outer side of a structure, you could say that it is anterolateral. If something were described to you as anteromedial, you would know that it was on the front and inner side of the body or body part.

TERMS COMPARING SIDES OF THE BODY

The language of medicine also has terms for indicating the side of the body, or of a body part, in reference to another side. That may sound confusing at first, but you will find that it is quite simple—and useful. For instance, suppose you are writing a report about a patient's arm, and you now want to report some findings about the leg that is on the same side of the patient's body. You can refer to the leg as the *ipsilateral* leg. The term ipsilateral means "on the same side as."

Next, suppose you want to report a finding concerning the patient's other arm, that is, the arm on the opposite side of the body from the arm you first examined. The term to use is *contralateral,* meaning "on the opposite side from." In other words, if you had first referred to the right arm, you would call the left arm the "contralateral arm" or the "contralateral upper limb."

Now that you have mastered the basic anatomic terms, we can start using them to learn about the structure, location, and function of the body's blood vessels.

CHAPTER REVIEW

- The three terms meaning that something lies or is moving in the direction of the head are cranial, superior, and cephalad.
- The two terms meaning that something is closer to the feet than to the head are caudal, or caudad, and inferior.
- The front half of the body is its anterior, or ventral, aspect. The back half is called the posterior, or dorsal, aspect.
- Medial means in the direction of the midline; lateral means in the direction away from the midline.
- The most commonly used directional prefixes are infra-, intra-, post-, supra-, inter-, sub-, and ante-.
- The term ipsilateral means on the same side as; the term contralateral means on the opposite side from.

SECTION TWO

The Blood Vessels

The vascular system does not consist only of a single kind of blood vessel. Instead, several different types of vessels work together as a "closed loop" of channels to distribute blood, and the substances and gases it carries, throughout the body. Before you can understand how this vascular system works, you will need to understand something about the blood vessels themselves, including both their similarities and their differences.

CHAPTER

3

The Blood Vessels

When people think of the blood vessels, they usually think of arteries and veins. In speaking of the function of these vessels, many people will say, "Arteries carry blood that has oxygen in it, and veins carry blood that doesn't have oxygen." Both ideas are partly true—and partly false.

TYPES OF BLOOD VESSELS

First of all, the human body has three categories of blood vessels, not two: the arteries, the veins, and the capillaries, and each of these categories has subdivisions. The fact that veins and arteries exist has been known to medicine for thousands of years. Unfortunately, the functional difference between these vessels was misunderstood until relatively recent times. For true understanding to occur, the existence and function of the capillaries had to be discovered.

Hippocrates, the Greek physician known as "the father of medicine," theorized that all human disease was related to disturbances of precious fluids in the body which he called the cardinal humors: blood, phlegm (mucus), choler (yellow bile), and melancholy (black bile). When we describe a hot-tempered person as choleric or a sad person as melancholy we are using words that go back to Hippocrates.

By the time of the Romans, the physician Galen made additional discoveries that led him to modify, but not discard, Hippocrates' humoral theory. Galen, who was personal physician to the Emperor Marcus Aurelius, was also chief surgeon to the gladiators. As such, he had considerable opportunity to examine dead and injured human bodies. Galen proposed that the arteries, which had been thought to carry only air, also carried blood (a radical concept at the time!). He was also able to demonstrate experimentally that the arteries and veins were connected in some fashion, although centuries would pass before Western physicians learned what this connection was.

Physiology, the science of body function, came a long way because of Galen, but he did make one rather large error. Galen thought that the veins were conduits carrying nutrients to the tissues, and that the arteries carried nutrient-depleted blood back to the heart. It would not be until the seventeenth century that the true pathway of circulation was discovered.

The person responsible for this discovery was a physician named William Harvey, who has often been called "the father of modern physiology." Harvey first publicly expressed his theories regarding the circulatory system in a lecture he gave in 1616. According to Harvey, blood started in the heart, went to the lungs to pick up oxygen, was carried out to the tissues via the arteries, and finally returned to the heart by way of the veins. In a paper he published in 1628, more than 350 years ago, he stated:

> I began to think whether there might not be a motion, as it were, in a circle. Now, this I afterwards found to be true and I finally saw that the blood forced by the action of the left ventricle [of the heart] into the arteries was distributed to the body at large and its several parts in the same manner as it is sent to the lungs. These points proved, I conceived it will be manifest that the blood circulates, revolves propelled and then returning from the extremities to the heart, and thus that it performs a kind of circular motion.

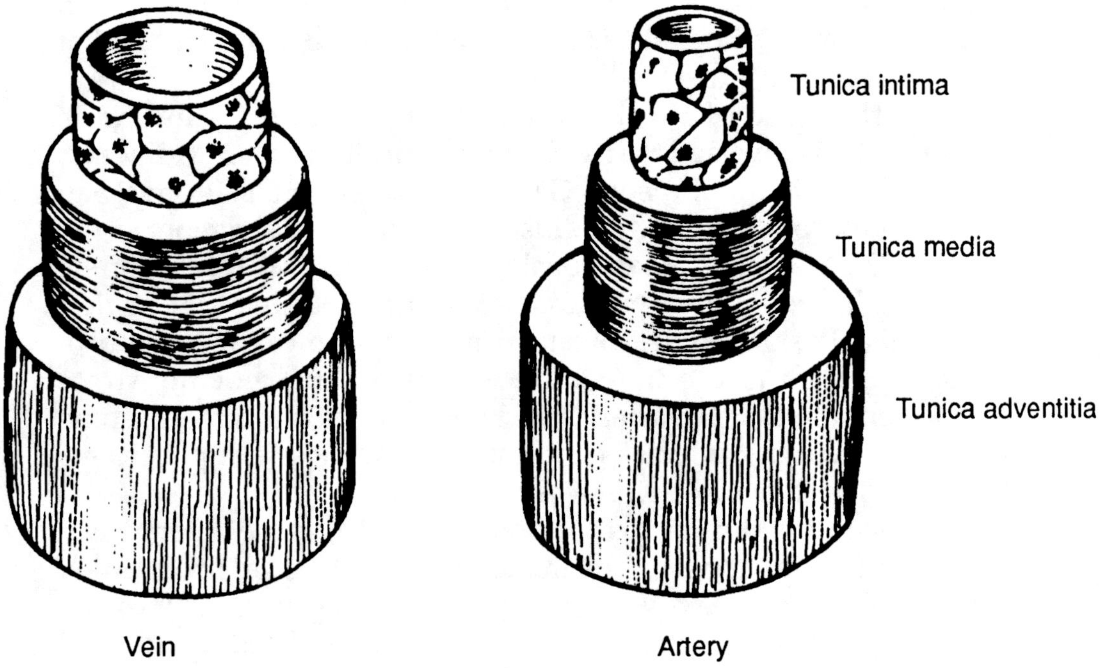

Figure 3.
The three layers of the vessel walls.

Unfortunately, William Harvey had no way of demonstrating that the circular motion he described actually occurred. For that reason, many anatomists and physicians rejected his concept.

Seventeenth-century medicine lacked a technology for viewing structures that could not be seen with the naked eye. The existence of the third type of blood vessel, the capillaries, was not discovered until after the development of the microscope. These tiny vessels form the connection between the arterial and venous systems and are the means by which the blood nourishes the tissues and carries away their wastes.

THE VESSEL WALLS

The vessels of the arterial and venous systems are basically tubes. The largest of these tubes have walls composed of three layers, or coats; the walls of the next largest consist of two of these coats; the walls of the smallest vessels consist of only one coat so thin it is composed of a single layer of cells. The layers are given the same names in both the arterial and venous systems, but their size, strength, and composition are somewhat different. (See Figure 3.)

The outermost layer of the vessel wall is called the *tunica adventitia*. Tunica is the Latin word for coat; adventitia is Latin for "extraneous" or "coming from abroad." A little trick for remembering the three vessel layers is to associate them with something familiar. So, think of someone who is adventurous as being outgoing, or brave enough to be on the outside, and you will find it easy to remember that the tunica adventitia is on the outside. Although "tunica adventitia" is the form most commonly used to describe the outside layer, some anatomy books use the term "tunica externa."

We are used to thinking of blood vessels as conduits that carry blood to or from other structures. However, blood vessels are composed of living tissue, so they also require nourishment. The adventitia of both veins and arteries is nourished by minute vessels called *vasa vasorum*, which means "vessels of vessels."

The middle of the vessel wall consists of a layer called the *tunica media*. The name of this layer is easy to remember. It comes from the same Latin root as the word medium, which means "in the middle." (Recall that medial refers to the midline of the body.)

The innermost layer of a blood vessel is called the *tunica intima*, coming from the Latin word for "within," intus. An easy way to remember the tunica intima is to think of an intimate

thought as one you keep deep inside; just so, the tunica intima is deep inside the vessel wall.

THE ARTERIAL SYSTEM

The Arteries

The largest vessels of the arterial system are the *arteries*. The tunica adventitia of the arteries is made up of very strong, white, fibrous tissue. It is so strong that it retains the shape of the vessel, keeping it from collapsing even when it is cut.

The tunica media of the arteries is a relatively thick layer sometimes called the muscle coat. In the largest arteries it is a combination of smooth muscle tissue, elastic tissue, and some white fibrous tissue. The expansion and contraction of this muscle coat helps maintain blood pressure and flow. The arterial vessels also need to be strong to withstand the pulsation caused by the pumping action of the heart, which begins before birth and continues until death, as much as ninety or a hundred years later.

The innermost layer of the artery, the tunica intima, is only one cell thick. It is composed of endothelial tissue, which is a specialized form of skin that lines body cavities. In normal arteries, the tunica intima provides a slick, waterproof lining for the vessel. (We do not tend to think of blood vessels as being waterproof, but if they were not, we would be in a lot of trouble!)

The Arterioles

Arteries begin as three-layered tubes supplying the major organs at the core of the body. As they divide into smaller and smaller branches toward the periphery of the body, they could be likened to winter vacationers traveling from Maine to Miami: They start out wearing many layers, but by the time they reach South Carolina they begin peeling off their coats. The adventitia begins to thin, then disappears altogether. Now the vessel, which consists of the tunica media, the tunica intima, and the hollow center, is called an *arteriole*.

One of the meanings for the suffix -<u>ole</u> is little, or small. By combining the suffix with the root of <u>artery</u>, you create a word that means "little artery." Again, as the arterioles reach the periphery, the tunica media begins to thin, then finally disappears altogether. Like travelers reaching Florida, the arteries have shed all but their innermost layer.

The Capillaries

You might think that the smallest arterial vessels would be called intimas, but instead they are called *capillaries*, from the Latin word for "hairlike." Actually, these tiny vessels are even smaller than hairs, too small to be seen with the naked eye. Not only are the capillaries small in diameter, but most are only about a millimeter long, or approximately 1/25th of an inch. Yet there are so many capillaries in the human body that someone once estimated that if they were laid end to end, the capillaries would form a chain 62,000 miles long. Another estimate that gives an idea of their vast numbers is that a single cubic inch of muscle tissue contains over 1.5 million capillaries.

With the discovery of capillaries, William Harvey's theory of circulation as a closed-loop system was finally validated. These tiny vessels are the link by which blood moves from the arterial to the venous system. This link occurs in complicated, tangled networks called *capillary beds*, or vascular beds, where the tiniest vessels enter arterial capillaries and emerge as venous capillaries. It is in the capillary beds found throughout the body tissues that oxygen and nutrients are supplied to the tissues. Carbon dioxide and other waste products of cellular metabolism are removed. The specialized structure of the intima permits this to take place.

Remember that the human body is composed of billions and billions of individual cells. Cells are organized into larger structures called tissues which, in turn, are organized into organs and organ systems such as the skin, the digestive system, the skeletal and muscular systems, and the circulatory system itself. The four categories of tissue are muscle, connective, nerve, and epithelial (skin).

Endothelial tissue, which is one of many specialized forms of skin, is composed of cells that resemble flat, overlapping scales. These cells are ideally suited to promote exchange of molecules, which is what occurs in the capillary beds.

The arterial system brings blood rich in oxygen and nutrients to the tissues. The job of the venous system is to return the blood, now laden with wastes and depleted of oxygen, to the appropriate organs to be cleansed and resupplied.

THE VENOUS SYSTEM

Beginning with the capillary beds, think of the venous system as the traveler starting back to Maine from Florida. A single layer of

clothing is sufficient in Miami, but as he moves north, our traveler must keep adding layers until he is bundled up enough to withstand the cold of Maine.

Leaving the capillary bed with their burden of waste products, the vessels are now called *venous capillaries,* since they are carrying venous, or "return" blood. Their walls of single endothelial cells enable them to absorb gases and chemicals into the blood they are carrying back, eventually, to the lungs and heart. When they acquire a second layer, the tunica media, they are called *venules,* or "little veins." Gradually, their structure comes to include a full outer coat, the tunica adventitia.

Although the three layers of the venous walls have the same names as those of the arteries, there are some differences in structure. Earlier, we said that the adventitia of an artery is strong enough to keep the vessel open, even if it is injured. In a vein, the adventitia is considerably thinner and much less strong. If you have ever tried to draw venous blood or start an intravenous infusion, you know that veins can collapse fairly easily.

The tunica media of the veins is also much thinner and weaker than an arterial media, and it contains far less elastic tissue. This makes sense: Arteries must withstand the beating of the heart, but veins are usually nonpulsatile. Consequently, they need less elasticity.

The venous tunica intima, like the arterial, consists of a single-celled endothelium. However, there is a major difference between it and the arterial tunica intima. That difference is a structure that was identified in 1574 by Aquapendente, the teacher of William Harvey: the venous valves. This long-ago physician also partially identified the function of the venous valves, that is, controlling the flow of blood. However, he believed that the veins carried blood <u>to</u> the tissues rather than <u>from</u> them, and therefore he thought the venous valves controlled blood flow from the heart rather than flow back to it.

The *venous valves* are also called <u>semilunar valves</u> because of their half-moon shape. They are formed by folds of the intimal epithelium and occur at intervals throughout the venous system. If you look at a venogram or a surgical or autopsy specimen of a vein, you will see periodic bulges, as though there were some kind of growth in the vein at those spots. If you were to cut the vein open along its length, you would find a valve in each bulging area.

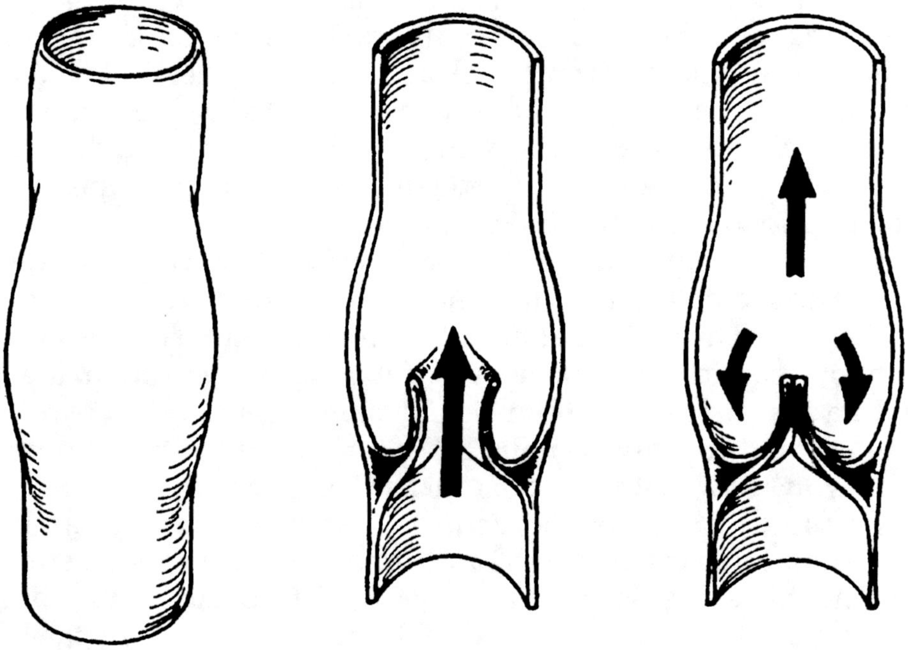

Figure 4.
Venous valves.

The distribution of these semilunar valves varies according to the area of the body, but all venous valves have two things in common. First, they are all designed to direct the flow of blood back toward the heart. Second, they are bicuspid, or two-cusped, valves (Figure 4).

The cusps are the flaps of tissue, or leaflets, that form the valve. As these leaflets open and close, they form pockets at the base of the valve which are called the *valvular sinuses.* (A sinus is a blind opening, or pocket, in a body structure.) The prefix bi- means two, or double; so a bicuspid valve is one in which there are two pockets, formed by two leaflets.

CHAPTER REVIEW

- Arteries, veins, and capillaries are part of a closed, continuous "loop" system in which blood travels from the heart and lungs, out to the periphery, and back to the heart.
- Arteries and veins, which branch to form arterioles and venules, are transport vessels; capillaries both transfer blood and promote exchange of blood gases and nutrients into and from tissues.
- Arteries and veins are nourished by internal vessels called vasa vasorum, "vessels of vessels."
- The walls of both arteries and veins are composed of three distinct layers called the tunica adventitia, the tunica media, and the tunica intima.
- The arterial tunica adventitia is strong enough to keep the vessel open even when it is severed or injured; the tunica media is a strong, elastic layer that allows the artery to pulsate throughout life.
- The tunica intima is only one cell thick and consists of endothelium, a specialized form of skin that lines body cavities.
- As arteries extend toward the periphery, the tunica adventitia becomes thinner and finally disappears altogether; beyond this point the now two-layered vessel is called an arteriole, or little artery.
- As the arterioles extend still further, the tunica media disappears, leaving single-walled vessels called arterial capillaries.
- Vessels entering the capillary bed are called arterial capillaries; as they leave the capillary bed they become venous capillaries.

34

- Venous capillaries gradually acquire a second layer, the tunica media, at which point they are called venules, or little veins.
- Venules gradually acquire a tunica adventitia and are then considered veins.
- Veins have bicuspid semilunar valves which direct the flow of blood back toward the heart.

Now, recall that at the beginning of this section we said that the statement that arteries carry oxygenated blood and veins do not is only partly true. This definition does not apply to the cardiopulmonary (heart/lung) circulation, which is discussed in Section III. The only definition that applies without exception to the blood vessels is that arteries always carry blood away from the heart, and veins always carry blood toward it.

SECTION THREE

The Cardiopulmonary and Systemic Circulations

In Section II you learned about the different types of blood vessels and the two "halves" of the circulatory system: arterial and venous. You learned that each of the major types of vessels had subdivisions: arteries, arterioles, and arterial capillaries in the arterial portion and venous capillaries, venules, and veins in the venous portion. So, too, can the entire circulatory system be divided into categories in a number of different ways. Each category may be called a "circulation," with all the categories together forming the circulatory system. For example, the *fetal circulation* is the system that nourishes and oxygenates the developing human. The term *hepatoportal circulation* refers to a specific pattern of blood flow involving the liver and the digestive organs. This circulation has not been the object of noninvasive testing until recently, when increasingly sophisticated techniques have enabled some noninvasive vascular laboratories to test aspects of it. Even so, the hepatoportal circulation remains outside the realm of the average vascular technologist or technician.

At present, the aspects of the circulatory system of specific interest to vascular technology are the *cardiopulmonary circulation* and the *systemic circulation*. The majority of this text is therefore devoted to these areas.

CHAPTER

4

The Cardiopulmonary Circulation

The *cardiopulmonary circulation* (from the Greek kardia, meaning heart, and the Latin pulmo, meaning lung) consists of the vessels that transport blood between the heart and the lungs. As already mentioned, the cardiopulmonary vasculature is the one exception to the "simple" definition of arteries as carrying oxygenated blood and veins as carrying unoxygenated blood. Once you understand the pattern of cardiopulmonary blood flow, you will see why that definition is not valid.

THE HEART

The heart is at the center of the vascular system: The arterial phase of the circulation begins there, and the venous phase ends there. Despite what the greeting cards and the poets would have us believe, the heart does not affect how we feel about someone, nor does it look like a valentine. The heart is really just a large muscle

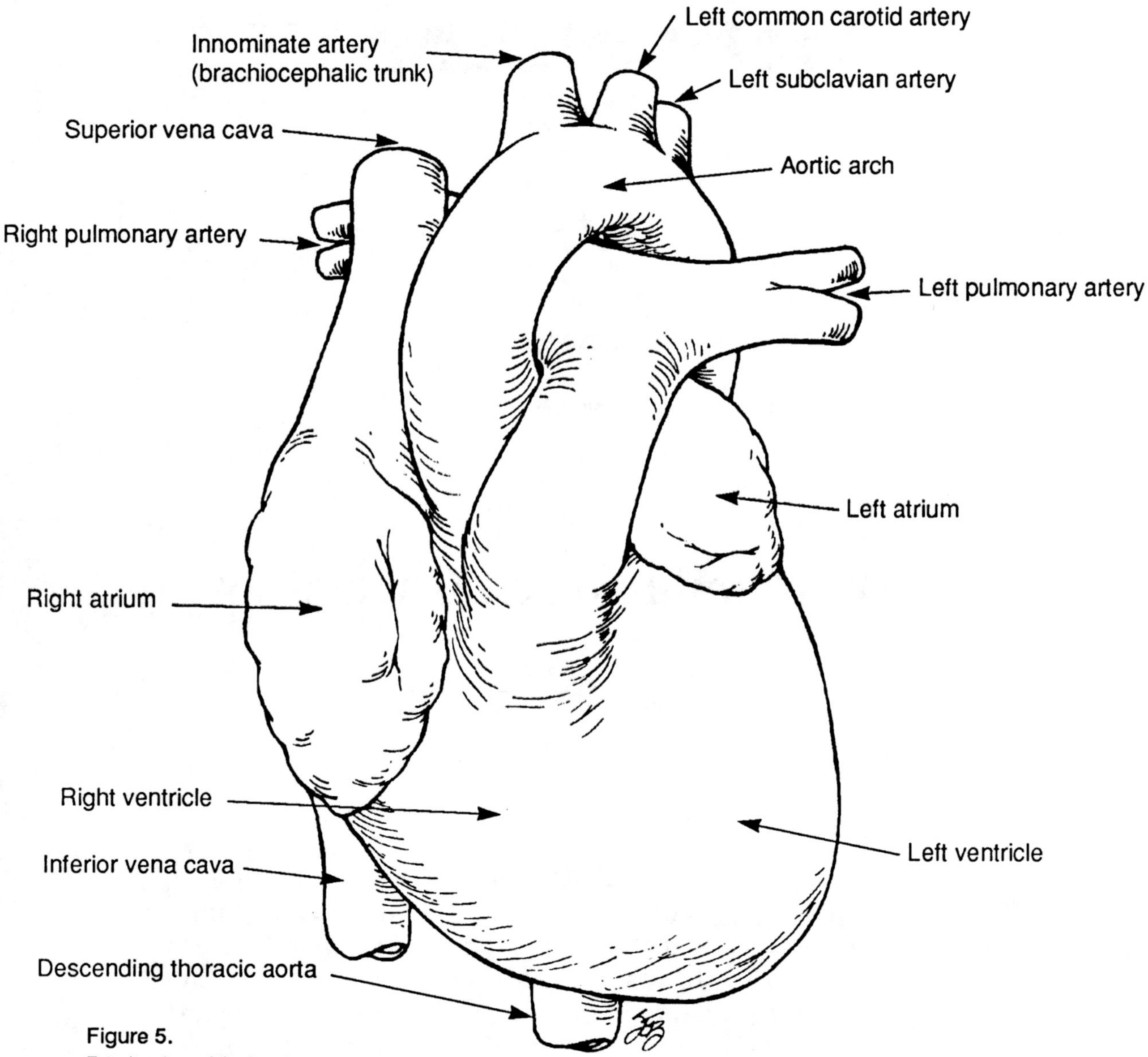

Figure 5.
Exterior view of the heart.

that serves as a pump. But even though the human heart may not be as pretty as a valentine heart, its function in the human body is crucial to life. Before we begin talking about the vessels of the cardiopulmonary circulation, we should look at the structure of the heart (Figure 5).

Location of the Heart

The heart lies slightly off-center in the thoracic, or chest, cavity. If you were to draw a vertical line through the middle of the body, separating it into right and left halves, you would find that roughly two-thirds of the heart is in the left half of the chest. The thoracic cavity is separated from the abdominal cavity by the diaphragm. The lower end of the heart, which is called the *apex cordis,* rests on the diaphragm.

Structure of the Heart

The heart of an adult is roughly the size of a man's closed fist. It is enclosed within a rather loose sac called the *pericardium.* This sac is composed of two layers: an outer protective covering of strong, white fibrous tissue, and an inner layer of smooth, moist serous (fluid-secreting) membrane, the *visceral pericardium.* This membrane folds back upon itself to form the parietal pericardium, also called the *epicardium,* which is the outermost layer of the heart muscle. Between these two layers is a small space called the *pericardial space.* It contains a fluid secreted by the serous membrane of the pericardium; this *pericardial fluid* acts as a lubricant, reducing friction when the heart beats against its protective sac.

Like the walls of the blood vessels, the wall of the heart has three layers: the epicardium, the myocardium, and the endocardium. Beginning from the outside, we first find the *epicardium,* the serous membrane that is continuous with the inner layer of the pericardial sac. The next layer, the *myocardium,* is composed entirely of muscle tissue (words beginning with my- or myo- refer to muscle tissue; mys is Greek for muscle). The myocardium forms the largest portion of the heart wall. Each of its contractions, or heartbeats, propels blood throughout the body. The *endocardium,* which lies on the inner aspect of the heart wall, is composed of a single layer of flat cells similar to those of the tunica intima that lines the blood vessels. (The prefix endo- means within.)

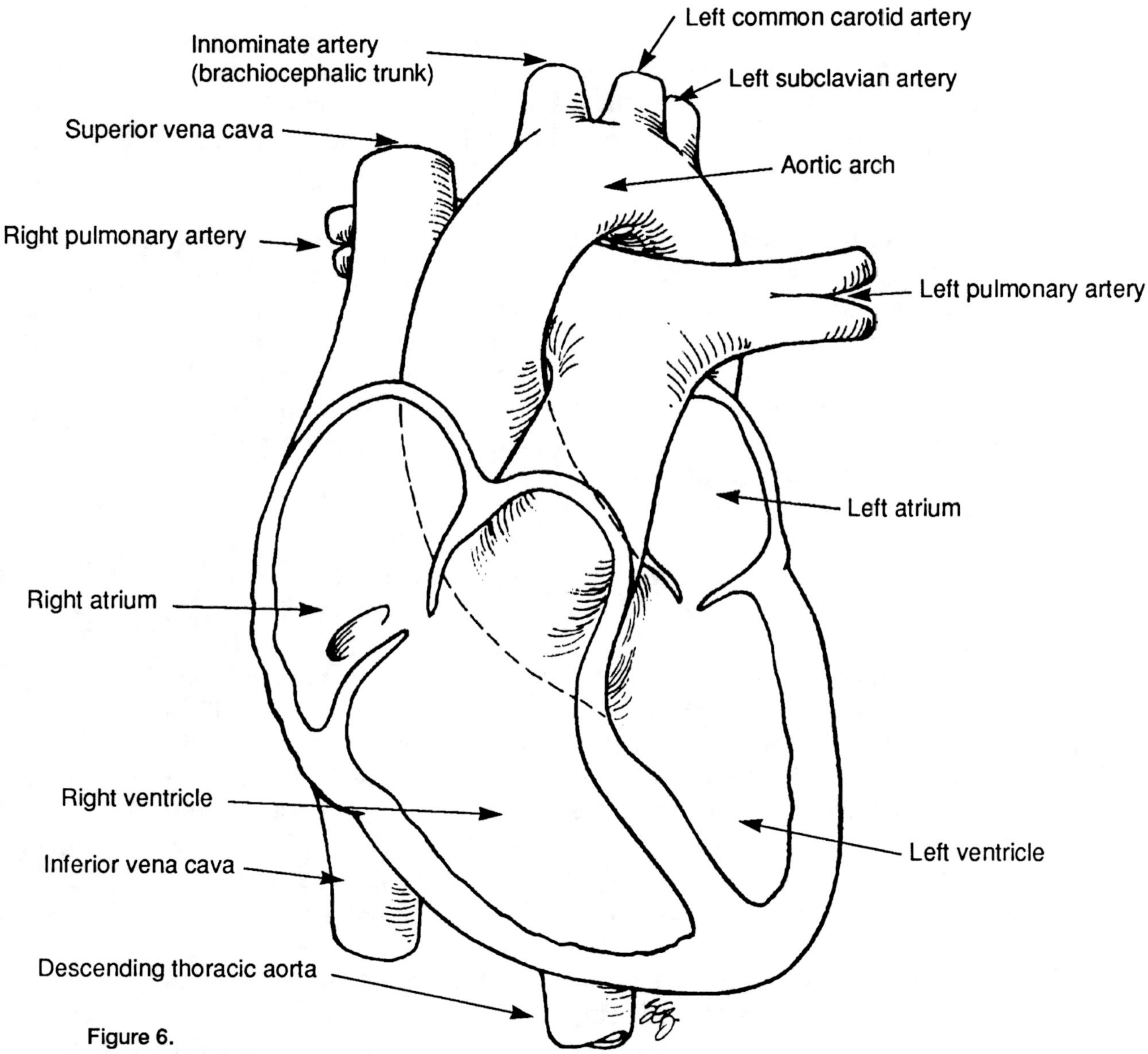

Figure 6.
Interior view of the heart.

The heart is divided into four cavities by membranous walls called septa (singular, septum; dividing walls within body cavities are generally called septa) (Figure 6). The right and left atria (singular, *atrium*) are at the top. The right and left *ventricles* are at the base. (In older texts, the upper chambers may be called "auricles"; however, this term is now used to refer only to the ear-shaped flaps that protrude from the atria.) The *interatrial septum* separates the right and left atria; the *interventricular septum* separates the right and left ventricles. The *atrioventricular* septum separates the atria from the ventricles. Blood passes through this septum by means of valves that are opened and closed by the expansion and contraction of the heart muscle. We will trace the flow of blood into, through, and out of the heart when we discuss the cardiopulmonary circulatory pattern.

Function of the Heart

Recall that the heart is a pump. The two atria are essentially collecting or holding chambers. Although they do pump, they must propel the blood only for a short distance. This requires relatively minor effort. The ventricles, on the other hand, take a very active role in the cardiac cycle, since they must pump to eject blood from the heart. For this reason, the ventricular myocardium is considerably stronger and thicker than the atrial myocardium. In addition, the right ventricle must pump blood only for a short distance, into the pulmonary artery. The left ventricle must pump blood to the farthest reaches of the body. Picture a seven-foot basketball player raising his arms to make a three-point shot, and you can appreciate the amount of work this ventricular pump must do! Therefore, the wall of the left ventricle, composed mainly of myocardium, is the thickest portion of the heart.

THE CARDIAC CYCLE

Blood flows into and out of the heart in a pattern called the *cardiac cycle*. This pattern repeats itself, over and over and over again, and in that sense it has no beginning or ending. However, we will begin our tracing of the cardiac cycle with the right atrium. The entire venous return of blood flows into this chamber from major veins called the venae cavae (see Chapter 7). This means that the blood in the right atrium is unoxygenated.

As both atria contract, the *tricuspid valve* between the right atrium and the right ventricle opens. (This valve derives its name

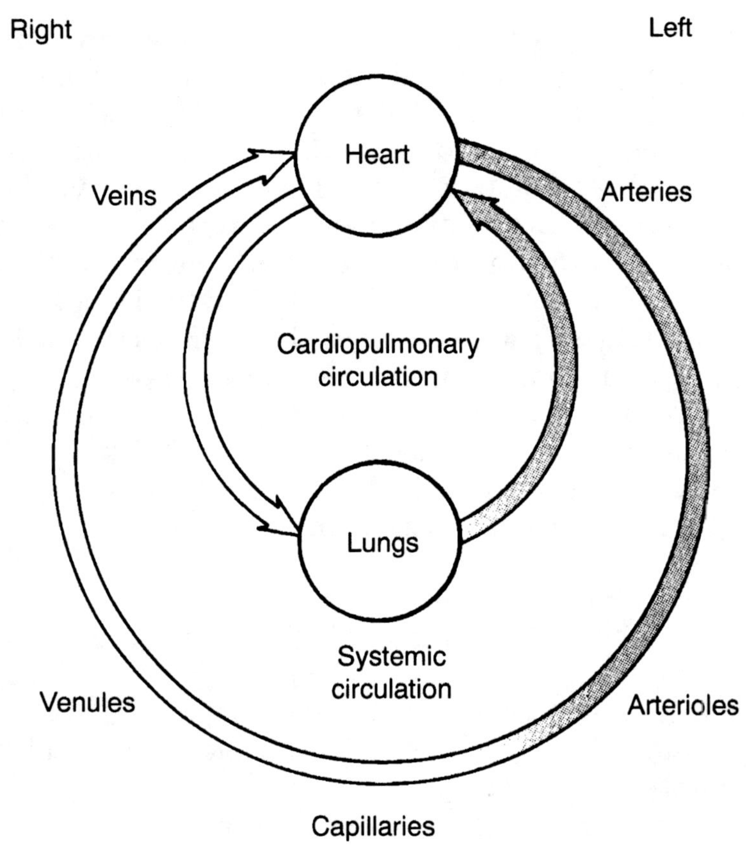

Figure 7.
Relationship of the systemic and cardiopulmonary circulations.

from its three leaflets, or cusps.) The unoxygenated venous blood drops into the right ventricle. Now the two ventricles contract, forcing the tricuspid valve shut and opening the *pulmonary semilunar valve* so that the blood can be propelled into the pulmonary arteries. These arteries transport the venous blood into the lungs so that it can be oxygenated once more. The flow of unoxygenated blood into the pulmonary arteries is one of the exceptions discussed in Chapter 3. These blood vessels are properly called arteries because they move blood away from the heart.

In the lungs, gas exchange takes place. Carbon dioxide, a waste product of cellular metabolism, is exchanged for oxygen. The oxygenated blood is then returned from the lungs to the heart by way of the pulmonary vein. This is the other exception: veins carrying oxygenated blood. Again, the pulmonary veins are named correctly because they carry blood back to the heart.

Oxygenated blood coming from the lungs through the pulmonary veins reenters the heart by filling the left atrium. As the left atrium contracts, this blood moves down into the left ventricle through the *mitral valve*. Because it has two flaps, the mitral valve is sometimes called the bicuspid valve of the heart. With the contraction of the ventricles, the cardiac cycle is complete. Oxygenated blood moves out of the heart through the aortic valve into the largest artery in the body, the aorta. (See Figure 7.)

This brief description greatly simplifies the complex activities of the heart and lungs. However, it should give you a general idea of how circulation in the body begins, and of how the cardiopulmonary circulation differs from the rest of the vascular system.

CHAPTER REVIEW

- The heart lies in the thoracic cavity, with roughly two-thirds of it in the left chest.
- The heart wall has three layers: the epicardium, the myocardium, and the endocardium. Most of the heart wall consists of myocardium.
- The heart has four chambers. The two upper chambers are the right and left atria; the two lower chambers are the right and left ventricles.
- The two atria are separated by the interatrial septum; the two

ventricles are separated by the interventricular septum. The atrioventricular septum divides the atria from the ventricles.

- Nonoxygenated blood passes through the tricuspid valves between the right atrium and the right ventricle, then through the pulmonary semilunar valves into the pulmonary arteries toward the lungs.
- Oxygenated blood returns to the heart from the lungs via the pulmonary veins. It enters from the left atrium and passes through the mitral (or bicuspid) valve into the left ventricle and from there out into the aorta.

CHAPTER

5

The Systemic Circulation: The Peripheral Arteries

This chapter discusses the vessels that make up the arterial network of the systemic circulation, with one exception. The arteries of the cerebrovascular network, which supply the head, are discussed in Chapter 6.

The systemic circulation contains many more peripheral arteries than are listed here. We will concentrate on (1) the vessels commonly considered to be the main arteries, (2) the arteries typically involved with the disease atherosclerosis and with noninvasive testing, and (3) information that is generally required for health professionals working in areas related to those topics. In addition to naming the arteries, we will also be looking at where they come from, where they go, what they do, and where they can best be palpated.

Palpation of an artery means using your fingers to feel the pulsation within the vessel—in other words, feeling its *pulse*. To feel a pulse, you push the artery against a firm structure within the

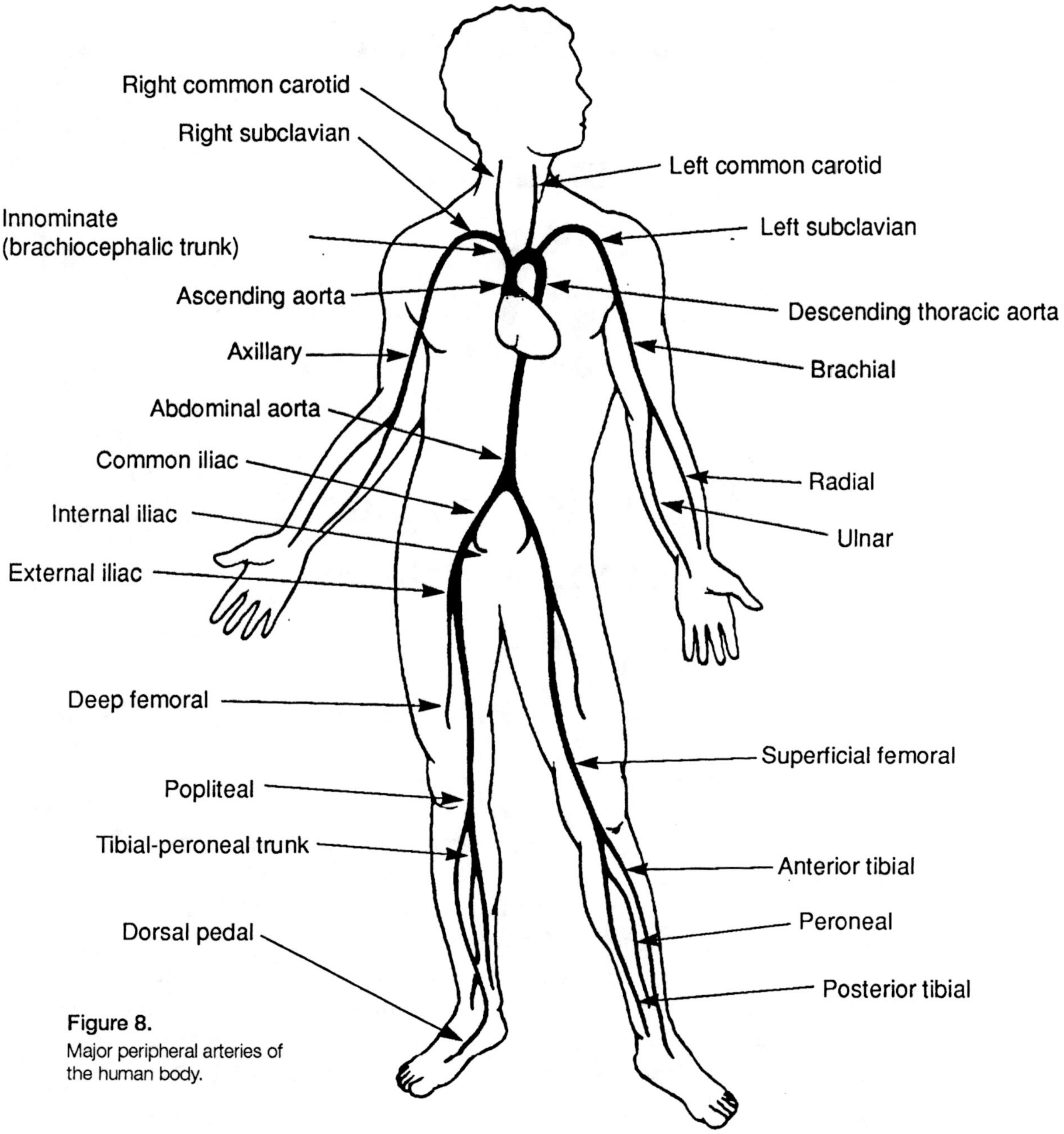

Figure 8.
Major peripheral arteries of the human body.

body against which it can beat. There are certain places where pulses can most easily be palpated, and these will be identified as we go along. In addition to giving landmarks for pulse sites, we will give you landmarks for remembering the location of an artery as it moves along its path. To provide an overall view, Figure 8 shows the major peripheral arteries of the human body.

In looking at the figure, and in reading the descriptions of arterial patterns, remember that blood vessels do not follow the precise "maps" provided in textbooks of anatomy. Each human body differs from others in a few ways or in many; consequently, blood vessel patterns vary from individual to individual. In any given patient, some vessels may not exist at all, some may start or end in unusual places, some may have branches that should exist, but do not, or that should not be there, but are. Each time an artery or vein is introduced, remember that when you are dealing with real people, you will find *anomalies*, or variations.

THE AORTA

Recall from Chapter 4 that the oxygenated blood entering the heart from the lungs moves out of the left ventricle and into the aorta. The *aorta* is the largest artery in the body, and all arterial distribution to the periphery begins here. All the other arterial vessels are branches and subbranches of the aorta, down to the smallest "twigs." Each division of the aorta divides into smaller arteries, and these in turn divide into still smaller arteries, and so on. If a vessel divides into two vessels, the point of division is called a *bifurcation*. If it divides into three, that point is called a *trifurcation*.

VESSELS SUPPLYING THE MYOCARDIUM

As it leaves the heart, the aorta initially travels upward in the thoracic cavity. Consequently, this portion of the aorta is usually called the *ascending* (rising) *aorta*. Although the term ascending thoracic aorta is sometimes used, "ascending aorta" is sufficient, because this is the only portion of the aorta that travels upward (cephalad, or toward the head).

The first branches of the aorta, the *coronary arteries*, arise from the ascending aorta. These are the vessels that supply the heart muscle (myocardium) itself. Clogging or blockage of these vessels leads to the condition we call a heart attack, which is more properly called *myocardial infarction* (MI). *Infarction* means the

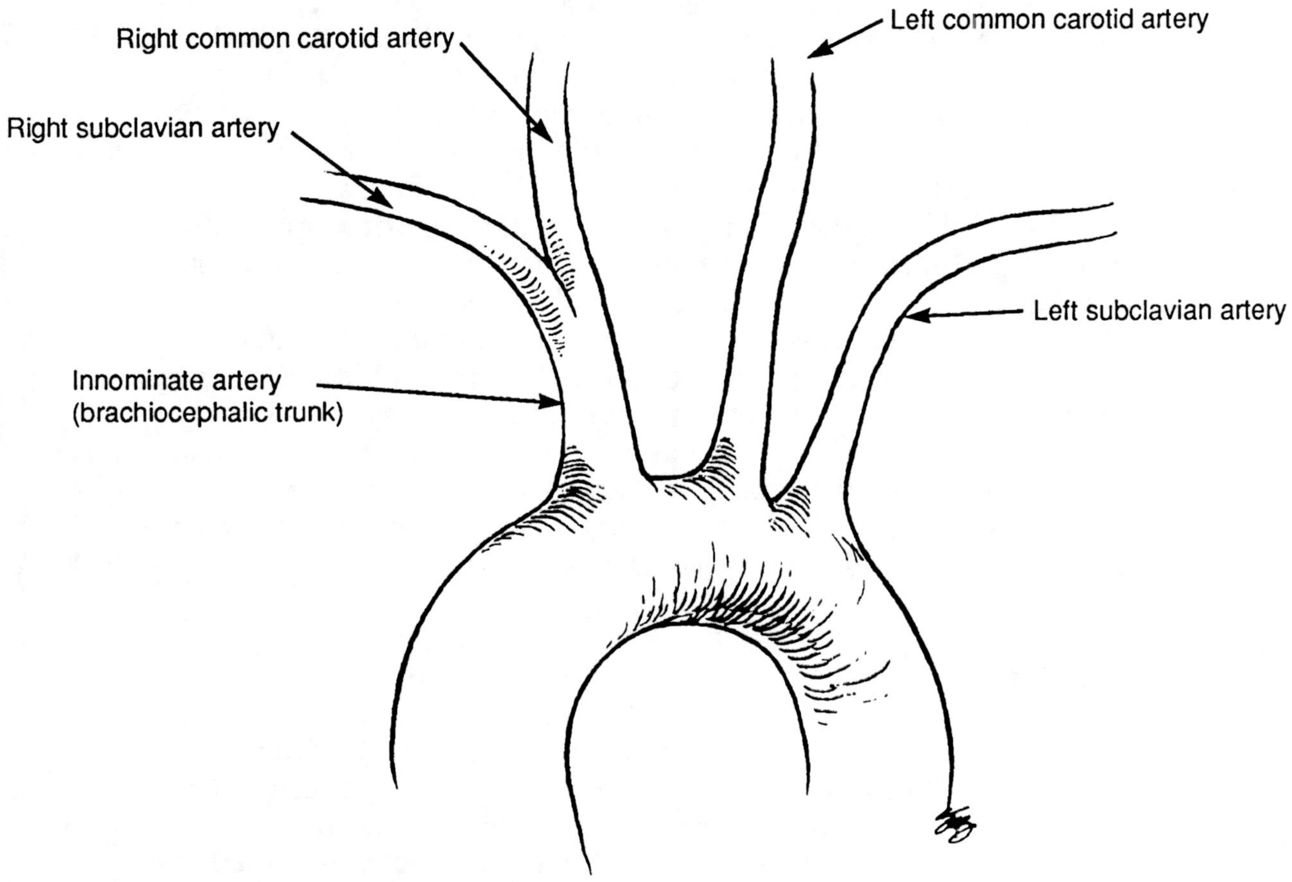

Figure 9.
The aortic arch and its branches.

death of tissue caused by deprivation of oxygen. Tissue receiving inadequate oxygen is said to be *ischemic;* if this condition is not corrected, the affected tissue will die.

After moving briefly upward, the aorta forms an arch near the top of the chest and begins moving downward. Three vessels normally originate in this portion of the aorta, which is called the *aortic arch,* or the arch of the aorta: the innominate (or brachiocephalic) artery, the left common carotid artery, and the left subclavian artery. These three arteries are sometimes called the *great vessels.* (See Figure 9.)

One of the names of the *brachiocephalic artery* tells you where its branches will go: brachio- means pertaining to the arm, and -cephalic means pertaining to the head. This artery branches into the right subclavian artery, which supplies the right upper extremity, and the right common carotid artery, which is one of the arteries supplying blood to the head. The carotid arteries are discussed in Chapter 7.

In most individuals, the second artery arising from the aortic arch is the *left common carotid artery.* The third is the *left subclavian artery,* which supplies the left upper extremity. The right and left subclavian arteries follow about the same course and serve the same function: supplying blood to the upper extremity.

BLOOD SUPPLY TO THE UPPER EXTREMITY

The Subclavian Artery

The first of the inflow, or supply, vessels for the upper extremity are the *subclavian arteries.* To simplify discussion, we will now drop the "left" and "right," because this circulation is essentially the same on both sides of the body. However, you should remember that each area discussed is approximately duplicated (allowing for individual anomalies) on the contralateral side.

Blood vessels usually are named for other structures in or near the same area of the body, most often bones. The clavicle, or collarbone, is the landmark for identifying the subclavian artery. To palpate the subclavian artery, it is usually easier to use an infraclavicular rather than a supraclavicular approach. (Recall that infra- means beneath or under; supra- means over or above.) The palpating fingers should move along the underside of the clavicle. It sometimes helps to start by visualizing the point where the right and left clavicles join, and the point where the shoulder attaches to the trunk. The subclavian pulse is often found about halfway between these two points.

The Axillary Artery

The subclavian artery travels laterally across the chest and then moves into the axilla, or armpit. Here its name changes to *axillary artery,* for the area of the body through which it travels. This artery can be easily palpated in the axilla.

The Brachial Artery

Moving out of the axilla and into the upper arm, or brachium, the axillary artery becomes the *brachial artery.* The "brachio-" in words used to refer to the upper extremity is taken from this portion of the upper extremity, which begins at the shoulder joint and ends at the elbow.

The landmark for palpating the brachial artery is the *antecubital fossa.* A fossa is a depression or hollowed space. If you bend your elbow, you form a hollow space on the ventral, or anterior, surface of your arm. Cubitus is the anatomic term for elbow. Thus, <u>ante</u>- plus <u>cubital</u> plus <u>fossa</u> means a space formed on the front of the elbow.

In the general area of the antecubital fossa, the brachial artery bifurcates to form two new vessels. This bifurcation may occur at, above, or below the elbow, depending on the individual body.

The Radial and Ulnar Arteries

The new branch that travels along the lateral side of the forearm is called the *radial artery* because it travels next to the radius bone. This artery is palpated at the anterolateral (anterior and lateral) aspect of the wrist. The other forearm bone is called the ulna, and it lends its name to the artery that travels along with it on the medial aspect of the forearm: the *ulnar artery.* The ulnar artery is also palpated at the wrist, but on the anteromedial (anterior and medial) side. People tend to be either "radial dominant" or "ulnar dominant," meaning that either the radial pulse or the ulnar pulse will be stronger without any disease being present.

Both the radial and the ulnar arteries branch several times and then are rejoined in the hand by two *palmar arches.* The names of these arches derive from their relative positions in the hand. In the normal anatomic position, with the palmar surface of the hand facing outward, the surface that is closer to the viewer is uppermost, or <u>superficial</u> to the other. The palmar arch in this position is called the *superficial palmar arch;* the arch that is deeper in the hand is called the *deep palmar arch.*

The superficial palmar arch is formed by an *anastomosis,* or joining, of the terminal portion of the ulnar artery with the palmar branch of the radial artery. The deep palmar arch is formed by an anastomosis of the terminal portion of the radial artery with the palmar branch of the ulnar artery. Therefore, you could also say that the radial artery terminates in the deep palmar arch and the ulnar terminates in the superficial palmar arch.

The Digital Arteries of the Hand

Coming off the superficial palmar arch are the *digital arteries,* which supply blood to the fingers. The digital arteries ramify, or branch out, into the arterioles and arterial capillaries that nourish the tissues in each digit.

In the hand, the digits are the fingers (in the foot they are the toes). You probably know them by their common names—thumb, index finger, middle finger, ring finger, and little finger or pinkie. More properly, the fingers are designated by numbers, starting with digit #1, the thumb. Thus digit #2 is the index finger, #3 the middle finger, #4 the ring finger, and #5 the little finger. This is how you would designate them if you were recording digital blood flow.

Each digit has both a lateral and a medial digital artery. These arteries are also sometimes referred to according to the artery in the forearm from which they receive their blood supply. The lateral digital artery of each finger would thus be called the *radial digital artery* (RDA), and the medial digital artery would be called the *ulnar digital artery* (UDA).

ARTERIES THAT SUPPLY THE TRUNK

Now that we have traced the path of the arteries supplying the upper extremity, we can return to the aorta to trace the pathway of blood supplying the major organs and other structures of the chest and abdomen.

Below the vessels that branch off at the aortic arch, the aorta moves downward in the thorax, or chest. From the aortic arch to the level of the diaphragm, this portion of the aorta is called the *descending thoracic aorta.* It has a number of branches that may be grouped, or classified, as visceral or parietal branches. *Visceral* is an adjective meaning that something is related to a viscus (plural, viscera), which is another name for a major organ within a body cavity. *Parietal* is an adjective that refers to the walls of a structure (a cavity or hollow organ, for example).

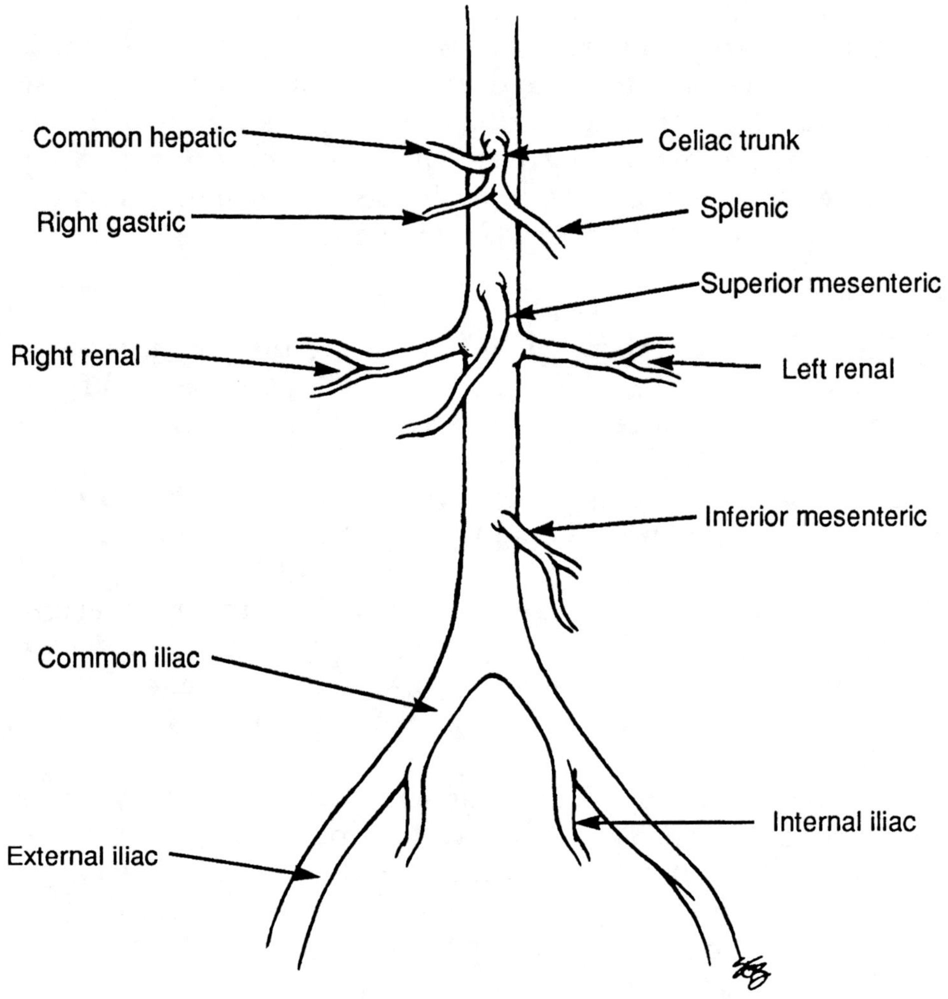

Figure 10.
Visceral branches of the abdominal aorta.

The visceral branches of the descending thoracic aorta supply blood to the pericardium, the mediastinum, the esophagus, and the bronchi. The parietal branches supply the thoracic side of the diaphragm, the chest muscles, and the mammary glands.

As the descending thoracic aorta passes through the diaphragm, it takes the name descending abdominal aorta or more simply, the *abdominal aorta*. In the abdomen, the aorta goes only downward, so "descending" is not necessary. A number of visceral and parietal branches come from the abdominal aorta.

The five *visceral branches* of the abdominal aorta are considered its major branches (Figure 10). They include:

- The celiac artery, sometimes called the celiac trunk or the celiac axis, which has three major branches,
- the superior mesenteric artery,
- the right and left renal arteries, and
- the inferior mesenteric artery (IMA).

The Celiac Artery (Celiac Trunk, Celiac Axis)

The *celiac* artery is a small artery that branches anteriorly almost straight out of the aorta. It trifurcates immediately into (1) the left gastric artery, (2) the common hepatic artery, and (3) the splenic artery. Although each of these branches actually supplies blood to more than one organ, the primary responsibility of each is to serve the organ for which it is named. The *left gastric artery* supplies the stomach (the root gastr- refers to the stomach); the *common hepatic artery* serves the liver (hepat- refers to the liver); the *splenic artery* serves the spleen.

The Superior Mesenteric Artery

The second major branch of the abdominal aorta is the *superior mesenteric artery* (SMA), which supplies blood to the small intestine and, to a lesser extent, the proximal portion of the colon. (The *mesentery* is the richly vascular lining of the bowel.)

The Renal Arteries

The third and fourth major branches of the abdominal aorta occur as a pair. The *right renal artery* and the *left renal artery* supply blood to the kidneys. (*Renal* means of or pertaining to the kidneys.)

The Inferior Mesenteric Artery

The last of the major branches is called the *inferior mesenteric artery*

(IMA). It is the primary source of blood for the large intestine (the colon), supplying the left half of the transverse colon, the descending colon, and most of the rectum.

By the way, the superior and inferior mesenteric arteries were not named that because of their relative size or importance. Although it is true that the diameter of the superior mesenteric artery is larger than that of the inferior mesenteric in most individuals, and that it generally carries more blood than the inferior mesenteric, that is not the reason for its name. The designations "superior" and "inferior" refer to the position of these arteries in relation to the renal arteries; the superior mesenteric artery lies above, or superior to them, and the inferior mesenteric artery lies below, or inferior to them.

The other visceral branches of the abdominal aorta supply blood to the ovaries or testes and to the suprarenal glands.

ARTERIES THAT SUPPLY THE LOWER EXTREMITIES

At approximately the level of the umbilicus, the abdominal aorta terminates by bifurcating into the *right* and *left common iliac arteries,* which take their name from the iliac, or hip, bone. These arteries are the beginning of the inflow distribution to the lower extremities. As we did for the arteries serving the upper extremities, we will discuss the iliac arteries and their branches in the singular, remembering that the patterns being described are approximately duplicated on the contralateral side.

The Internal Iliac (Hypogastric) Artery

The common iliac artery has two branches. The branch that goes inward and begins the blood supply to the organs of reproduction is called the *internal iliac artery* or, alternatively, the *hypogastric artery.*

In the male, the internal iliac artery becomes the *internal pudendal artery,* which trifurcates into the three vessels supplying the penis: the *superficial dorsal,* the *deep cavernosal,* and the *spongiosal arteries.* (Each takes its name from the region of the penis it supplies: the dorsum, the corpus cavernosum, and the corpus spongiosum.) In the female, the internal pudendal portion of the internal iliac artery trifurcates into the *deep artery of the clitoris,* the *dorsal artery of the clitoris,* and *the artery of the bulb of the urethra.*

In both the male and the female, the internal iliac (hypogastric) artery supplies the pelvic viscera (including the

lower rectum), the buttocks, and the medial aspect of the upper thigh.

The External Iliac Artery

Beyond the point where the internal iliac (hypogastric) artery branches off, the common iliac artery is known as the *external iliac artery*. It continues the progression of blood to the lower extremity. As it passes from the area of the iliac bone and enters the region of the femur, or thigh bone, its name reflects this changing location. It is now called the *common femoral artery*, which can usually be easily palpated at the inguinal ligament.

A good general rule to remember when palpating pulses is that the more superficial (closer to the skin) the artery, the lighter your touch should be, and the deeper the artery, the heavier your touch should be. Since the common femoral artery lies deep within the groin, it takes a fair amount of pressure to palpate it properly, even though it is normally a large artery with a strong pulse.

The Common Femoral Artery (Profunda Femoris)

From the groin, the common femoral artery then continues into the proximal thigh, where it gives off a branch called the *deep femoral artery*, or *profunda femoris*. (Profunda is Latin for deep; when we call someone a profound thinker, we mean that person thinks deep thoughts.) The common femoral artery is sometimes referred to as "the artery of the thigh," because its function is to provide blood to the areas and structures within the thigh, such as the muscles and the hip joint.

The Superficial Femoral Artery

The continuation of the femoral artery, after the profunda branches off, is called the *superficial femoral artery* (SFA). The superficial femoral artery is sometimes referred to as "the artery of the leg," because its only role is to provide blood to the remaining portion of the lower extremity.

From the bifurcation of the abdominal aorta, all the vessels named have had more than one destination. The common iliac artery sent blood to both the internal iliac artery, which serves the pelvis, and the external iliac artery, which goes to the lower extremity. The external iliac artery, which becomes the common femoral artery, also has a branch that terminates before it reaches the leg (recall the definition of "leg" as extending from the knee to

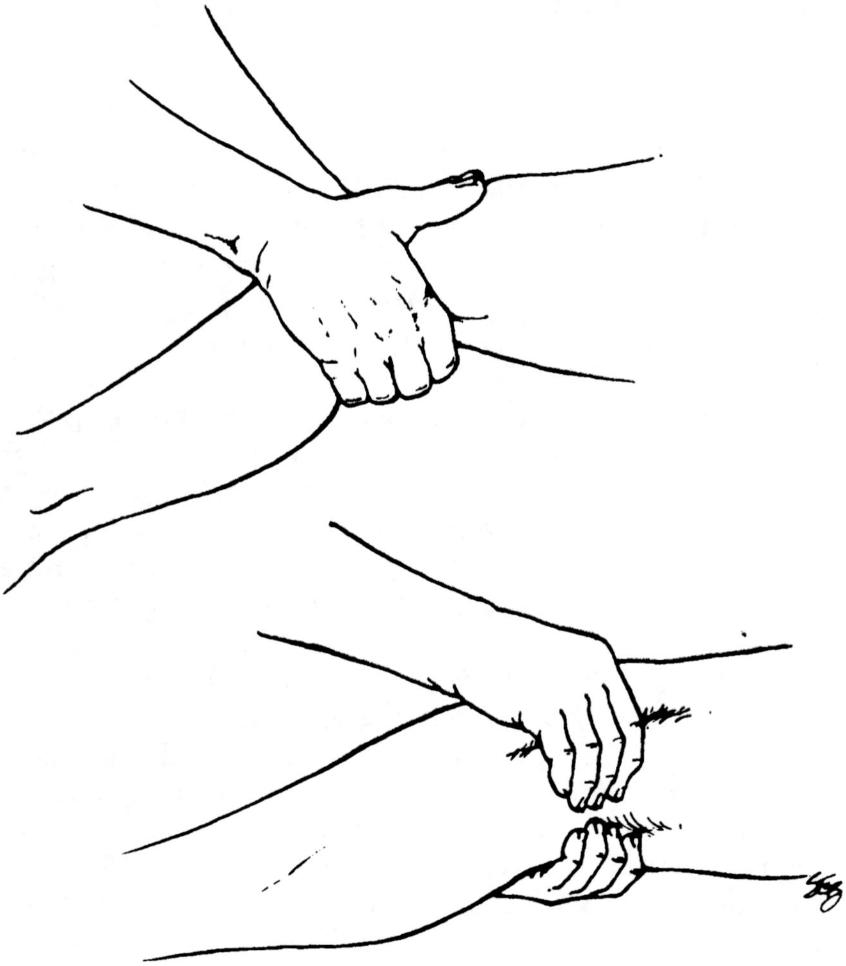

Figure 11.
Palpation of the popliteal arterial pulse.

the ankle). But the superficial femoral artery and its branches serve only the leg.

The pathway for the superficial femoral artery is the *adductor canal,* sometimes called Hunter's canal. Imagine the thigh as being trisected vertically; you will find a tunnel-like depression running up and down the middle portion. This is the adductor canal, which contains the femoral blood vessels, both artery and vein, as well as the saphenous nerve. This canal is your landmark for locating the superficial femoral artery.

The Popliteal Artery

As the superficial femoral artery passes into the area behind the knee called the *popliteal fossa,* its name changes to *popliteal artery.* The popliteal arterial pulse is very difficult for many people to learn to palpate. It is generally easier to do this by standing next to and facing the patient as he or she lies supine.

1. Use the bony base of your hands to hold the leg, grasping it just below the knee joint on either side and bending the knee slightly as you do so. The patient's limb should be relaxed and slightly bent, and your fingers should be free (Figure 11).
2. Starting with either your right or your left hand, place the flat portion of your fingertips against the popliteal fossa just below the midpoint.
3. Press in smoothly and try to "roll" the artery against the tendons at the side of the fossa.
4. If you cannot find the pulse, release your fingers and try the same technique with your other hand.

Do not be discouraged if you cannot find the artery quickly. The key to palpating all pulses, but especially the popliteal pulse, is practice.

The Tibial Arteries

Below the popliteal fossa, the popliteal artery is said to trifurcate, although the branching is more like a double bifurcation. The arteries formed by this branching, the anterior tibial, posterior tibial, and peroneal arteries, are often collectively referred to as the *trifurcation* or *infrapopliteal arteries.*

First, the popliteal artery divides into a larger branch called the *anterior tibial artery* (ATA) and a smaller one called the *tibial-peroneal trunk.* The anterior tibial artery takes its name from the *tibia,* the larger of the two leg bones and the one that bears weight. The other leg bone is the *fibula.* To remember which is which, think of a fib as a "little lie" and the fibula as a "little leg bone." The anterior tibial artery passes in front of (anterior to) the tibia and then swings up onto the foot at the ankle. Here it takes a new name, the *dorsalis pedis artery* (DPA). Pedis is Latin for foot, so the dorsalis pedis is the one located on the dorsal surface of the foot.

Returning to the trifurcation of the popliteal artery, we can now trace the course of the tibial-peroneal trunk. Very quickly, this vessel bifurcates into the posterior tibial and the peroneal arteries.

The *posterior tibial artery* (PTA), like the anterior tibial artery, takes its name from its relationship to the tibia. In this case the artery runs behind (posterior to) the bone, rather than in front of it. It also terminates at the foot, but instead of being at the front of the ankle, the landmark is at the side of the foot. The posterior tibial artery is palpated slightly behind and below the *medial maleolus,* or inner ankle bone.

The Peroneal Artery

The remaining trifurcation vessel is the *peroneal artery,* which is named by the Greek, rather than the Latin, name for the fibia. The Greek word for this bone, which the Romans called the fibia, was perone. The peroneal artery moves through the deep muscle compartment on the posterolateral aspect of the leg. Near the ankle, it bifurcates into an anterior and a posterior branch. The anterior peroneal artery may often be palpated on the foot slightly in front of and above the lateral malleolus, or outer ankle bone.

The anterior peroneal pulse is usually much more difficult to palpate than the dorsalis pedis or the posterior tibial pulse. It is important to remember the rule about palpating pulses: The deeper the artery, the firmer the pressure; the closer to the skin the artery is, the lighter the touch. If you used as much pressure while palpating the dorsalis pedis as you did for the common femoral artery, you would "wipe out" the pulse altogether.

The Digital Arteries of the Foot

Like the hand with its palmar arch, the foot also has an arch structure. This is called the *plantar arch* and is formed by the

Table 1.
Major peripheral arteries: origins, locations, pulse sites.

ARTERY	ORIGIN	LOCATION	PULSE SITE
Aorta, abdominal	(continuation of) descending thoracic aorta	abdomen	upper medial umbilical region
Aorta, ascending thoracic	left ventricle	thorax	N/A
Aorta, descending thoracic	(continuation of) aortic arch	thorax	N/A
Aortic arch	(continuation of) ascending thoracic aorta	thorax	N/A
Artery of the clitoral bulb	internal pudendal a.	clitoris	N/A
Axillary	(continuation of) subclavian a.	axilla	axilla
Brachial	(continuation of) axillary a.	arm	antecubital fossa
Brachiocephalic (innominate)	aortic arch	thorax	N/A
Carotid, left common	aortic arch	neck	left side of neck, as low as possible
Carotid, right common	(bifurcation of) brachiocephalic a. (innominate a.)	neck	right side of neck, as low as possible
Cavernosal, deep	internal pudendal a.	penis	penis
Celiac	abdominal aorta	abdomen	N/A
Clitoral, deep	internal pudendal a.	clitoris	N/A
Clitoral, dorsal	internal pudendal a.	clitoris	N/A
Digital, lower extremities	plantar arch	toes	lateral & medial aspects of the toes
Digital, upper extremities	superficial palmar arch	fingers	lateral & medial aspects of the fingers
Dorsal, superficial	internal pudendal a.	penis	penis
Dorsalis pedis	anterior tibial a.	foot	dorsal aspect of foot
Femoral, common	(continuation of) external iliac a.	groin	inguinal ligament
Femoral, deep (profunda femoris)	common femoral a.	proximal thigh	N/A
Femoral, superficial	(continuation of) common femoral a.	thigh, along the adductor canal	mid medial thigh
Gastric	celiac a.	abdomen	N/A
Hepatic	celiac a.	abdomen	N/A
Hypogastric (internal iliac)	common iliac a.	abdomen	N/A
Iliac, common	(bifurcation of) abdominal aorta	abdomen	N/A
Iliac, external	(continuation of) common iliac a.	abdomen	N/A
Iliac, internal (hypogastric)	common iliac a.	abdomen	N/A
Innominate (brachiocephalic)	aortic arch	thorax	N/A
Mesenteric, inferior	abdominal aorta	abdomen	N/A
Mesenteric, superior	abdominal aorta	abdomen	N/A
Palmar arch, deep	(anastomosis of) radial & ulnar arteries	hand	N/A
Palmar arch, superficial	(anastomosis of) ulnar & radial arteries	hand	N/A
Peroneal	(bifurcation of) tibial-peroneal trunk	posterolateral leg	lateral malleolus
Plantar arch	(anastomosis of) anterior & posterior tibial arteries	foot	N/A
Popliteal	(continuation of) superficial femoral a.	dorsal knee area	popliteal fossa
Profunda femoris (deep femoral)	common femoral a.	proximal thigh	N/A
Pudendal, internal	internal iliac a.	abdomen	N/A
Radial	(bifurcation of) brachial a.	lateral forearm	anterolateral wrist
Renal	abdominal aorta	abdomen	N/A
Splenic	celiac a.	abdomen	N/A
Spongiosal	internal pudendal a.	penis	penis
Subclavian, left	aortic arch	clavicular area of thorax	mid left infraclavicular region
Subclavian, right	(bifurcation of) brachiocephalic a. (innominate a.)	clavicular area of thorax	mid right infraclavicular region
Tibial, anterior	(bifurcation of) popliteal a.	anterior aspect of the leg	anterior, distal leg; proximal to the ankle
Tibial, posterior	(bifurcation of) tibial-peroneal trunk	posteromedial leg	medial malleolus
Tibial-peroneal trunk	(bifurcation of) popliteal a.	leg	N/A
Ulnar	(bifurcation of) brachial a.	medial forearm	anteromedial wrist

anastomosis (joining) of the terminal branches of the anterior and posterior tibial arteries. The *digital arteries* of the foot arise from this arch. Like the fingers, the toes have both a lateral and a medial artery. Also like the fingers, the toes are numbered, with the great toe being #1 and the little toe being #5.

A summary of the major peripheral arteries, their origins, locations, and pulse sites appears in Table 1.

CHAPTER REVIEW

- The main vessel leaving the heart is the aorta, which has four regions: the ascending thoracic aorta, the aortic arch, the descending thoracic aorta, and the descending abdominal aorta.
- The coronary arteries arise from the ascending aorta.
- The three great vessels that normally arise from the aortic arch are the innominate, or brachiophalic; the left common carotid; and the left subclavian.
- The innominate/brachiophalic artery bifurcates to form the right subclavian and the right common carotid arteries.
- Even though the right and left subclavian arteries have different origins, once formed, they have virtually identical routes.
- The pathway of blood flow in the upper extremity is subclavian to axillary, brachial bifurcating to form radial and ulnar, radial and ulnar joining via the deep and superficial palmar arches, and palmar arches giving rise to lateral and medial arteries in each digit.
- The five visceral branches of the abdominal aorta are the celiac artery (which gives off the gastric, hepatic, and splenic arteries), the superior mesenteric artery, the right and left renal arteries, and the inferior mesenteric artery.
- The blood flow path in the lower extremity (excluding branches to the groin, etc.) is the common iliac to the external iliac; the external iliac to the common femoral; the common femoral to the superficial femoral; the superficial femoral to the popliteal; the popliteal to the anterior tibial (ultimately the dorsalis pedis), the posterior tibial, and the peroneal (collectively the infrapopliteal vessels); and the infrapopliteal vessels joining to form the plantar arch, from which arise the lateral and medial arteries of the digits.

CHAPTER

6

The Systemic Circulation: The Cerebral Arteries

Before we begin discussing the individual arteries of the cerebrovascular circulation, we need to define a pair of important terms. Cerebral arteries are often described as being intracranial or extracranial. *Intracranial* means within the cranium, or skull, and *extracranial* means outside the skull. Some of the cerebral vessels are exclusively intracranial, some are exclusively extracranial, and others have portions located in each area.

THE COMMON CAROTID ARTERIES

To learn about the cerebrovascular portion of the systemic circulation, we need to go back to a structure we discussed in Chapter 5: the aortic arch. Remember that in most individuals, the branching pattern at the aortic arch forms three arteries: the innominate, or brachiocephalic artery; the left common carotid artery; and the left subclavian artery. We have already followed the

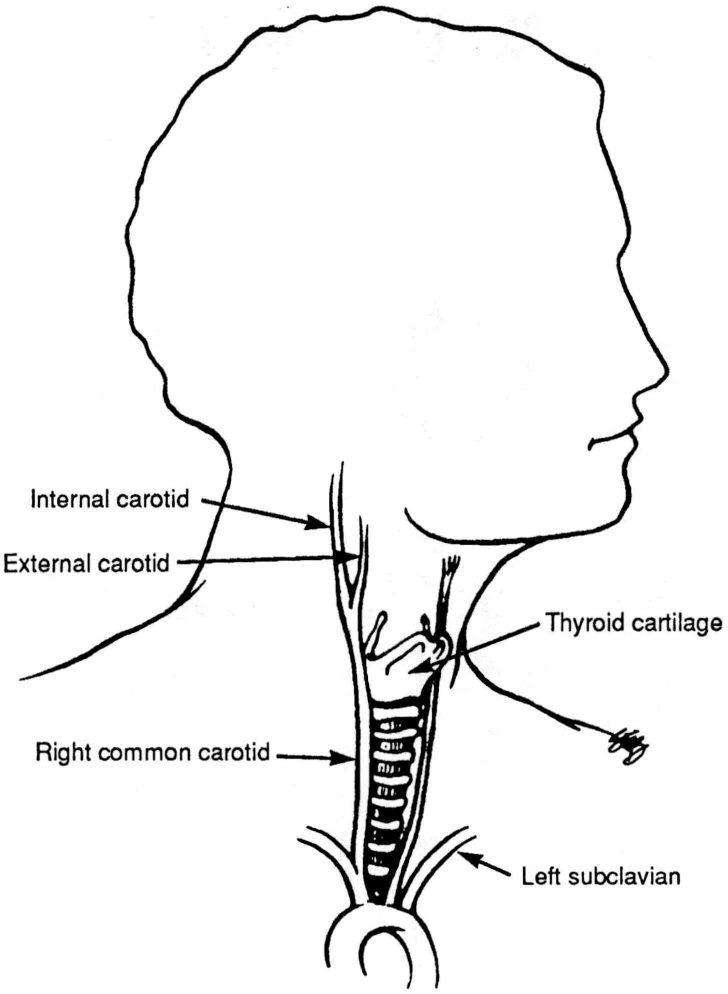

Figure 12.
Bifurcation of the common carotid artery.

subclavian arteries to their termination; now we will go back and talk about the remaining branches of the aortic arch, the common carotid arteries.

Like the right and left subclavian arteries, the right and left common carotid arteries originate from different sources but follow approximately identical patterns after that. The *right common carotid artery* (CCA) originates at the bifurcation of the innominate, or brachiocephalic, artery. The *left common carotid artery*, on the other hand, usually arises directly from the aortic arch. This difference in point of origin can make a difference in the ease with which each of the common carotid pulses is felt. Since the right common carotid has its origin closer to the level of the clavicle, it is usually somewhat easier to palpate than the left common carotid, which starts closer to the heart.

Now that we have discussed the origin of both common carotid arteries, we can stop specifying which is being described, since their pattern is the same bilaterally (on both sides of the body).

The common carotid arteries move in a fairly straight path upward in the neck on either side of the trachea (the windpipe). At the top of the trachea is a structure called the *larynx*, or voice box. The larynx is formed by nine different pieces of cartilage, the largest of which is called the *thyroid cartilage*. Along with the fat pad that lies over it, the thyroid cartilage forms what is commonly called the Adam's apple. (Despite its name, both women and men have an Adam's apple.)

The common carotid artery usually bifurcates into its two terminal branches at the level of the thyroid cartilage. Since the entire common carotid artery lies within the neck, it is completely extracranial. It is also *cervical*, meaning that it lies in the neck. Either way of referring to it is correct.

Before tracing the path of the two branches of the common carotid artery, we need to cover some considerations involving the area where it bifurcates.

THE CAROTID BULB (CAROTID SINUS)

Look at Figure 12 carefully, and you will see that the common carotid artery does not merely divide at its bifurcation; it seems to be larger at that spot. This enlarged area is called the *carotid bulb*, or *carotid sinus*. Extremely pressure-sensitive nerve cells called *pressoreceptors* are located within the walls of the carotid sinus.

These pressoreceptors play a very important role in regulating the heart rate. (We will be talking more about regulation of the heart rate in Chapter 11, Mechanisms of Control.)

Stimulation of the carotid pressoreceptors causes *reflex bradycardia*, a reduction of the heart rate (the prefix brady- means slow or slowing). There are certain times when it is important to induce rapid, radical slowing of the heart rate. For example, in a condition known as paroxismal atrial tachycardia (PAT), the heart rate can suddenly jump to well over 150 beats per minute, more than twice the normal resting rate. To return it to more normal speed, a physician may use a technique called carotid massage, rubbing or massaging the carotid sinus to induce reflex bradycardia.

Consider, though, what might happen if pressure on the carotid sinus induced reflex bradycardia when the heart had been beating at a normal rate. Blood flow to the brain would be dangerously reduced. In fact, this is why people lose consciousness when they are being strangled.

Physical stimulation of the carotid sinus may also induce a type of heartbeat called premature ventricular contraction (PVC). Frequent episodes of PVCs can lead to ventricular tachycardia (tachy- means fast), then ventricular fibrillation, and then to asystole, the absence of any heartbeat.

One final point about the carotid bulb. Atherosclerotic plaque, the fatty deposit that clogs arteries, often accumulates at this point. Rubbing over the carotid bulb can dislodge a fragment of plaque, causing an embolus (a moving blood clot or other plug) that can lodge in the brain, possibly causing a stroke.

What do all these unpleasant possibilities have to do with our discussion here? Well, they have to do with palpation of pulses. There is only one safe place to palpate a common carotid arterial pulse, and that is as low in the neck as possible. Not everyone's carotid bulb occurs right at the thyroid cartilage. In some people the bifurcation lies very high; in others it occurs at a much lower level in the neck. So, to avoid stimulating the carotid sinus, it is important to remember to palpate for the common carotid as close to the clavicle as possible.

THE CAROTID "FAMILY"

The common carotid artery has no branches in the neck. It terminates at its bifurcation, becoming two arteries, the internal

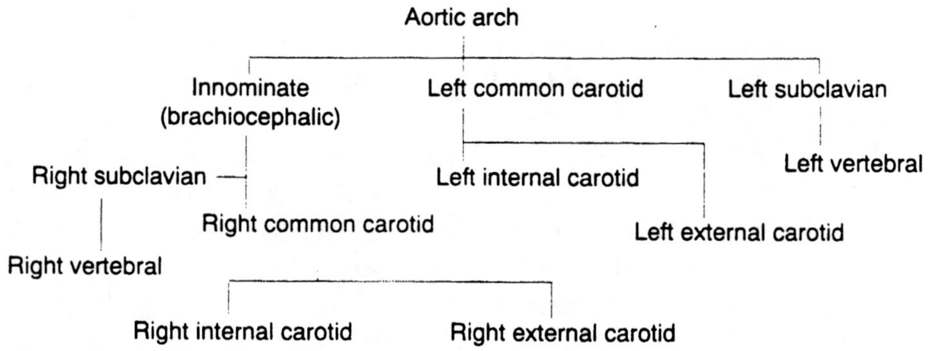

Figure 13.
Origin and progression of the carotid family of arteries.

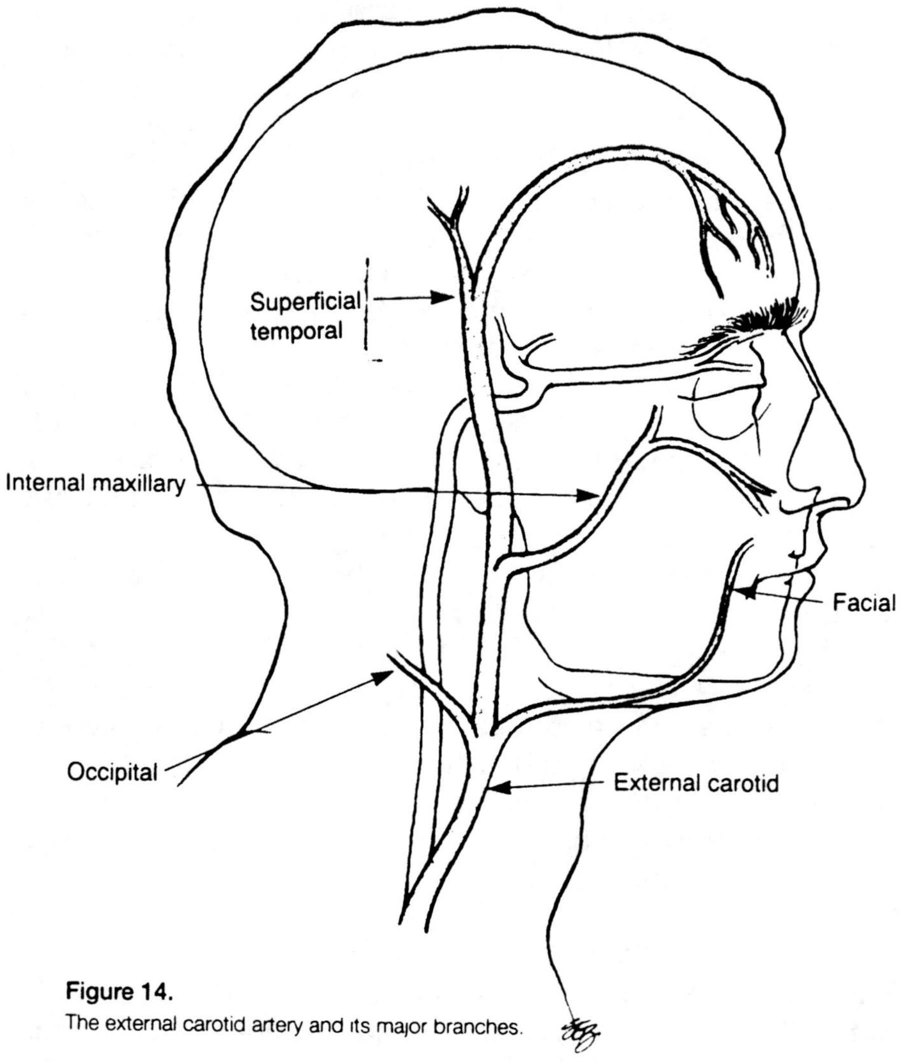

Figure 14.
The external carotid artery and its major branches.

and external carotid arteries. The *internal carotid artery* is called "internal" because it ultimately enters the skull and provides blood to the main internal structure of the skull, the brain. The *external carotid artery*, for the most part, supplies blood to extracranial structures such as the scalp and the skin. For a "family tree" showing the origin and progression of the carotid "family," refer to Figure 13.

With this background, we can explore the terminal branches of the carotid artery, beginning with the external carotid artery (Figure 14).

THE EXTERNAL CAROTID ARTERY

The external carotid artery (ECA) has a great many branches, the first of which arises shortly after the external carotid forms. A complete listing of these branches is in Table 2, but for practical purposes we will concentrate on the more major branches that are directly or indirectly involved with noninvasive testing.

The Occipital Artery

At approximately the level of the lower jawbone, or mandible, the external carotid gives off a branch called the *occipital artery*. It derives its name from the occiput, the part of the skull at the base of the head. The occipital artery passes behind the ear and distributes blood to the branch vessels that supply the muscles of the neck and scalp and other external structures in the area.

The Facial Artery

At just about the same level, the external carotid artery has another branch called the *facial artery*. It swings forward under the jaw and then moves up onto the face just in front of the masseter muscle.

If you were to find the midpoint on an imaginary line from the cleft of the chin to the end of the mandible near the earlobe, you would be in a good spot to begin your search for the best palpation site for the facial artery. Using a light touch, since this is a superficial artery, try to "roll" the artery against the jawbone from the top. Or, to use some of the medical terminology you learned in Section I, place your fingers in a supramandibular position for palpation of the facial arterial pulse.

The facial artery gives off a number of small branches as it moves across the cheek, or buccal, area toward the medial, or inner, aspect of the eye, where it terminates as the *angular artery*.

Table 2.
Branches of the external carotid artery.

ARTERY	MAJOR BRANCHES
Ascending pharyngeal	inferior tympanic a. posterior meningeal a.
Facial (external maxillary)	angular a. ascending palatine a. inferior labial a. superior labial a.
Internal maxillary (maxillary)	anterior tympanic a. buccal a. deep auricular a. deep temporal a.'s descending palatine a. inferior alveolar a. infraorbital a. masseteric a. middle meningeal a. posterior superior alveolar a. pterygoid canal a. sphenopalatine a.
Lingual	profunda linguae a. sublingual a.
Occipital	
Posterior auricular	stylomastoid a.
Superficial temporal	middle temporal a. transverse facial a. zygomaticoorbital a.
Superior thyroid	superior laryngeal a.

The Internal Maxillary Artery

The next branch of the external carotid artery is the *internal maxillary artery* (IMA). "Internal" should not be taken to mean that this artery goes inside the skull. It does, however, travel through the bony prominences of the face. It takes its name from the *maxilla,* or upper jaw.

The internal maxillary artery is very complicated, with many branches, and it is not externally palpable. One important branch of this artery is the *middle meningeal artery,* which arises from the internal maxillary artery deep within the area of the muscles of mastication (chewing). The middle meningeal artery passes upward and becomes an intracranial vessel by entering the skull through an opening called the foramen spinosum. *Foramen* is a word we will be using several times in this chapter. It refers to a natural opening or passage through a body part, usually bone. The *foramen spinosum* is an opening in the sphenoid bone, which is in the ventral portion of the cranial floor and which forms part of the floor and walls of the orbit (eye socket).

The *meninges,* from which the middle meningeal artery takes its name, are the membranes that cover the brain and spinal cord: the dura mater, pia mater, and arachnoid. The middle meningeal artery provides blood to the dura mater (the outermost of the meninges) and to the cranial bones. Like the internal maxillary artery from which it branches, the middle meningeal artery cannot be palpated.

The internal maxillary artery continues to move anteriorly and medially until it finally terminates by entering an opening in the cheekbone called the *infraorbital foramen,* which means the "under-the-eye-socket opening." As the internal maxillary artery emerges from the intraorbital foramen onto the face, it becomes the *infraorbital artery* (IOA).

The infraorbital artery is small, with a pulse that is difficult to palpate. The pulse may be found on the upper cheekbone, under the eye socket (the orbit), usually near the middle of the eye. It requires a very light touch in palpation.

The Superficial Temporal Artery

After the external carotid artery has given off the internal maxillary artery, it ceases to be called the external carotid. From that point on, it becomes the *superficial temporal artery* (STA). This artery passes in front of the ear as it moves superiorly on the head,

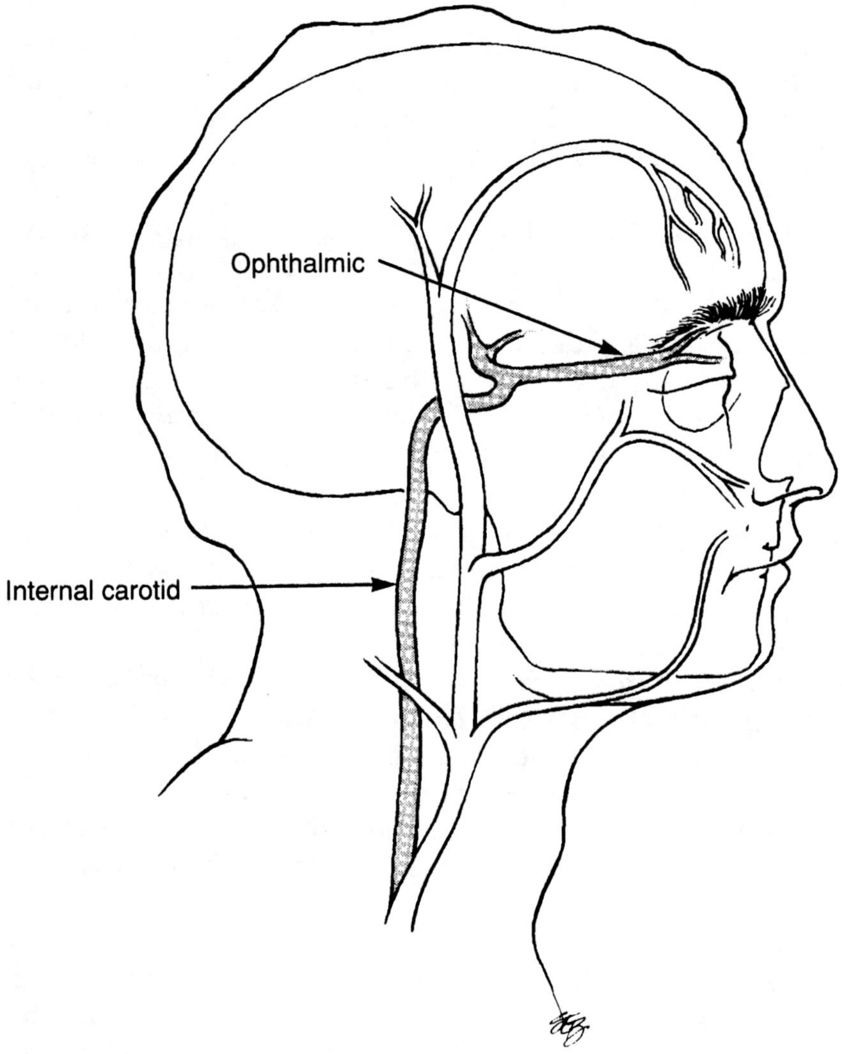

Figure 15.
The internal carotid artery and its first branch.

onto the temple area, finally terminating by ramifying on the forehead.

When we say that an artery is *ramifying,* we mean that it branches out, or terminates into its endpoint vessels. So, the superficial temporal artery terminates by filling the capillary bed of the forehead. This is an important point to remember, as we will see later in this chapter.

There are two places where you can easily palpate the superficial temporal pulse. The first is the little hollow spot you can feel just in front of the opening of the ear canal. The other spot is higher, on the temporal bone itself. By the way, this is the artery you can sometimes feel when you are trying to sleep on your side and it seems as though there is a pounding in your forehead.

THE INTERNAL CAROTID ARTERY

Unlike the external carotid artery, the *internal carotid artery* (Figure 15) has no branches in the neck at all. Instead, it moves superiorly as a single vessel until it enters the cranium. The internal carotid artery is the only one of the three carotid arteries that has a dual nature; it has both an extracranial and an intracranial portion.

The extracranial or cervical (neck) portion of the internal carotid artery begins at the bifurcation of the common carotid and terminates where the internal carotid enters the skull. It does so by passing through small holes on each side of the foramen magnum called the *carotid canals.* The *foramen magnum* is the large central opening through which the spinal cord enters the cranium. Once it passes through these canals, the internal carotid artery becomes an intracranial vessel.

Inside the skull, it continues to move upward, not straight but along a series of curves that swing first anteriorly, then medially, and then posteriorly. From the side, it resembles the bottom half of the letter "s." This curved portion of the internal carotid artery is called the *carotid siphon,* from the Greek word meaning a bent tube of unequal length. You can see this formation under your own bathroom or kitchen sink.

The Ophthalmic Artery

At this point, the internal carotid artery gives off its first branch, the *ophthalmic artery* (see Figure 15). Since ophthalmos is the Greek word for eye, it is logical to assume that the ophthalmic artery supplies the eye, which it does. It moves anteriorly toward the eye,

giving off many branches that supply the eye itself, as well as the eye socket and adjacent structures. The three terminal branches of the ophthalmic artery, which exit onto the face, are used in a noninvasive test called the periorbital Doppler examination or, sometimes, ophthalmosonometry. These three branch vessels can be easily palpated around the eye.

Beginning at the side (laterally) and moving toward the center (medially), the first of these terminal branches is the *supraorbital artery* (SOA). It swings over the eyeball and leaves the orbit, or eye socket, at the top, above the eye (hence, supraorbital artery). It then passes onto the forehead through the *supraorbital foramen*, an opening in the frontal bone (which you may know as the brow bone).

If you feel your own frontal bone along the eye socket, you should feel a small notch in the bone, as though someone had whittled it out. That notch is the supraorbital foramen, and if you palpate lightly above that point, you should be able to feel the supraorbital arterial pulse. This vessel is close to the skin and requires a very light touch. The supraorbital artery terminates by ramifying on the forehead.

Moving medially, the next terminal branch of the ophthalmic artery is the *frontal artery*. This artery also moves along the top of the orbit and exits onto the forehead, only it does so much closer to the inner aspect of the eye. To palpate the pulse of the frontal artery, feel lightly on the brow bone near the medial edge of your eyebrow.

The last and most medial of the ophthalmic artery's terminal branches is the *nasal artery*. It is similar in one way to the supraorbital and frontal arteries, but it also has a significant difference. It is the same in that it comes directly off the ophthalmic artery and swings out of the orbit at the circumference of the eye. However, instead of moving onto the forehead, it exits almost straight out of the orbit toward the bridge of the nose, where it terminates as the *angular artery*.

Like the branch of the external carotid known as the superficial temporal artery, the two temporal branches of the internal carotid ramify in the forehead. This means that if significant disease should block one of the branches of the carotid arteries, the potential for a collateral route exists. *Collateral circulation*, also called compensatory circulation, is an alternative route that develops through anastomosis (joining) of vessels when

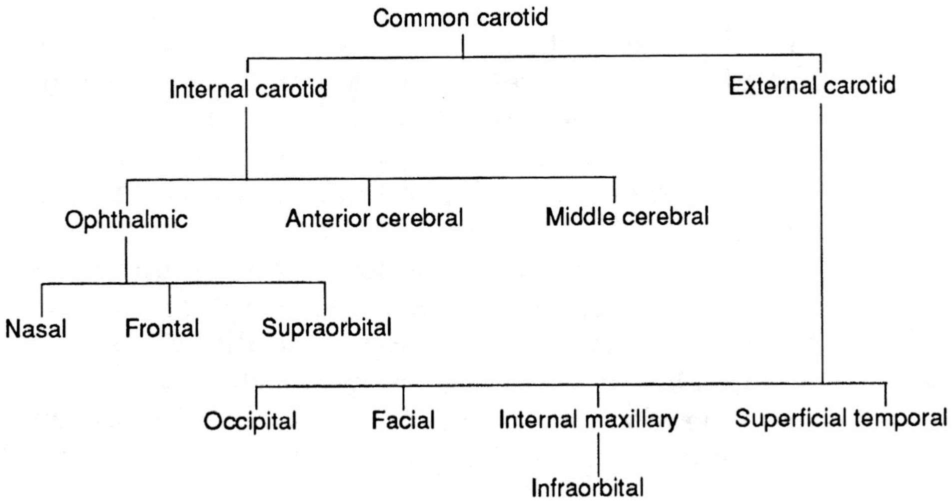

Figure 16.
Specific members of the carotid family of arteries.

an existing circulatory route is blocked or cut off. If one of the branches of the internal carotid artery were to become occluded (blocked), for example, the ipsilateral external carotid artery could readily extend itself by way of the supraorbital or frontal artery, to provide an alternative pathway.

In addition, the angular artery, which is the termination of the facial artery, ramifies in the same area as the nasal artery, providing yet another potential anastomosis between the circulatory pathways of the internal and external carotid arteries. Finally, the middle meningeal artery can anastomose with the ophthalmic artery to provide a fourth collateral route. These external-to-internal carotid pathways are all considered extracranial collateral routes. Later in this chapter you will see some possibilities for intracranial collateral routes.

The Anterior and Middle Cerebral Arteries

Beyond the point where the ophthalmic artery branches off, the internal carotid artery moves superoposteriorly and gives off a second branch called the *anterior cerebral artery.* From this point the internal carotid is called the *middle cerebral artery.* Another way of thinking of this is that the internal carotid artery bifurcates to form the anterior and middle cerebral arteries. Or, that the anterior cerebral and middle cerebral arteries are the terminal branches of the internal carotid artery.

Since the internal cerebral artery, like the others we have been discussing, occur on both the right and the left sides, it stands to reason that there would be right and left anterior cerebral arteries and right and left middle cerebral arteries. The right and left sides of the cerebrovascular circulation are connected by a small arterial vessel called the *anterior communicating artery,* which joins the right and left anterior cerebral arteries. If you put all seven of the vessels we have just identified together, you would have half of a circular formation called the circle of Willis.

The major branches of the second half of the carotid "family tree," which consists of the vessels just discussed, are shown in Figure 16.

THE CIRCLE OF WILLIS

The *circle of Willis* is located at the base of the brain and is the source of arterial blood that nourishes and oxygenates this vital organ. It is an extremely important structure, both in health and

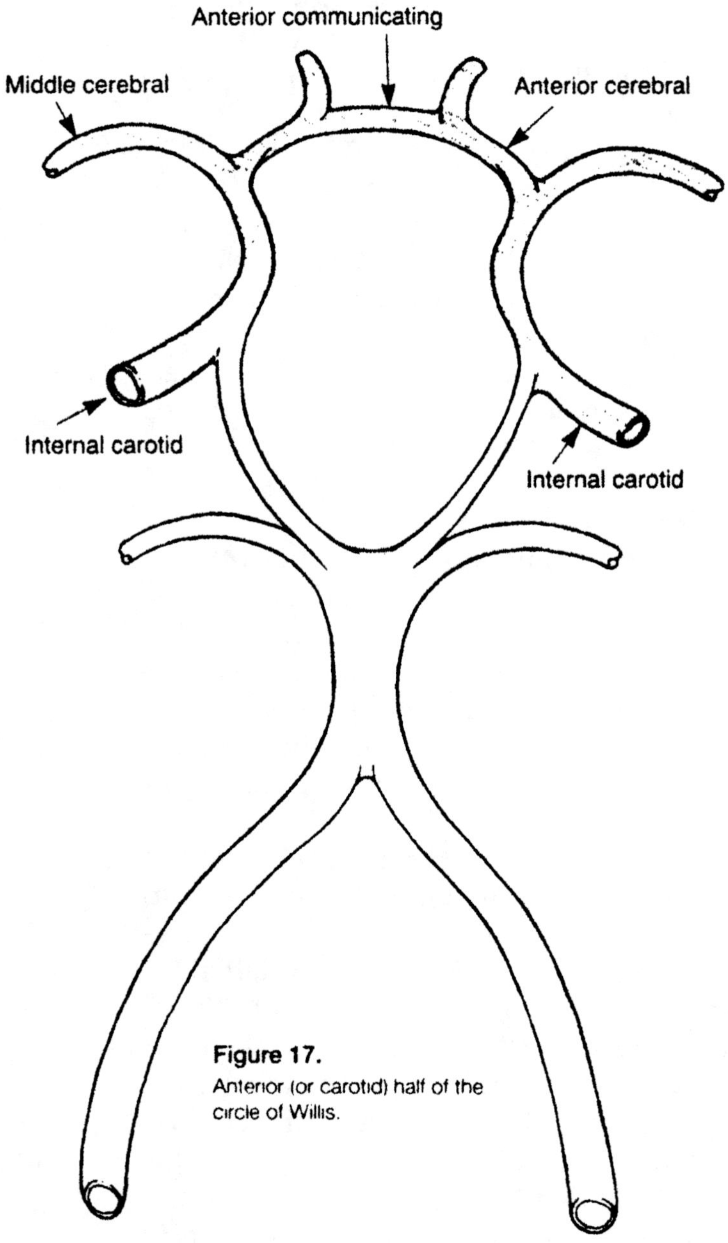

Figure 17.
Anterior (or carotid) half of the circle of Willis.

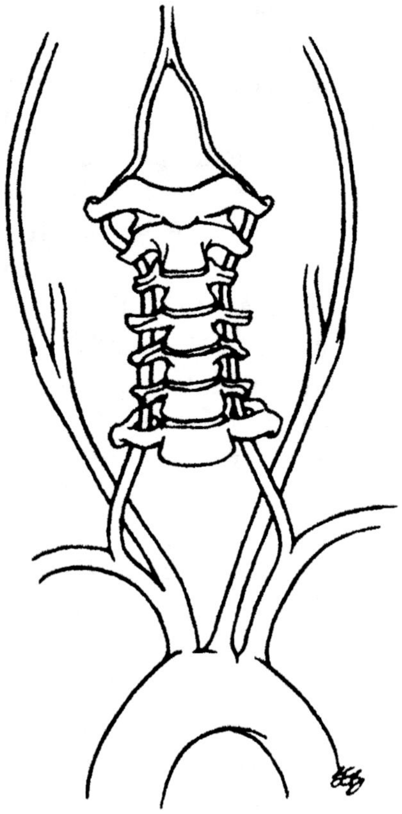

Figure 18.
The vertebral artery within the transverse foramina of the cervical vertebrae.

when carotid disease is present. Its front, or anterior, half consists of the vessels we have been describing (Figure 17):

- the right and left internal carotid arteries,
- the right and left anterior cerebral arteries,
- the right and left middle cerebral arteries, and
- the single anterior communicating artery.

To construct the other half of the circle of Willis, we must start again from the aortic arch.

Recall that the first artery arising from the aortic arch in most individuals is the innominate, or brachiocephalic, artery, which bifurcates to form the right subclavian and the right common carotid arteries. The third of the arch vessels is normally the left subclavian artery. Now, we have already talked about where the subclavian artery goes, and we have just finished discussing the carotid arteries. What is left? The first branch of the subclavian artery.

The first branch of the subclavian artery is called the *vertebral artery*. It is named for the vertebrae, the bones of the spine. From its origin, the vertebral artery moves superoposteriorly toward the cervical vertebrae (the vertebrae that form the neck). Vertebrae have lateral bony projections called *transverse processes*, each of which has an opening called the *transverse foramen* (plural, foramina). The vertebral artery passes through the transverse foramen on its way to the skull (Figure 18), which it enters by passing through the foramen magnum along with the spinal cord. Once it passes through the foramen magnum, the vertebral artery is intracranial. Like the internal carotid artery, the vertebral artery has both extracranial and intracranial segments.

Inside the cranium, the right and left vertebral arteries join to form a single artery called the *basilar artery*. The basilar artery bifurcates to form the right and left posterior cerebral arteries. Coming off these vessels are the *right* and *left posterior communicating arteries*, which join, or communicate with, the internal carotid arteries. Thus, the most common configuration of the posterior half of the circle of Willis consists of:

- the right and left vertebral arteries,
- the basilar artery,

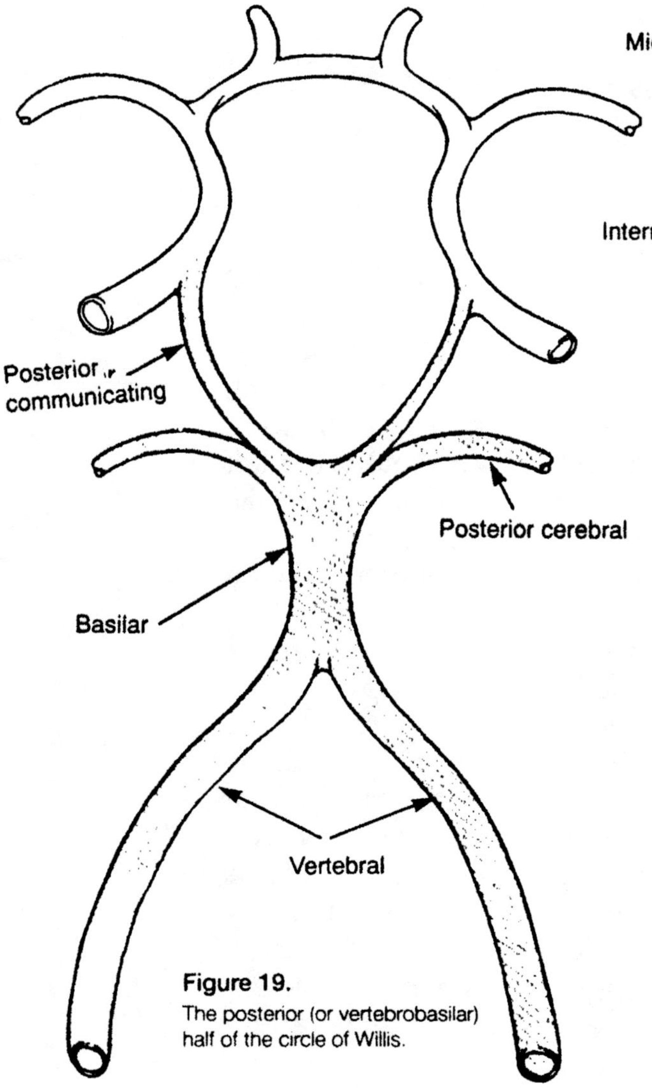

Figure 19.
The posterior (or vertebrobasilar) half of the circle of Willis.

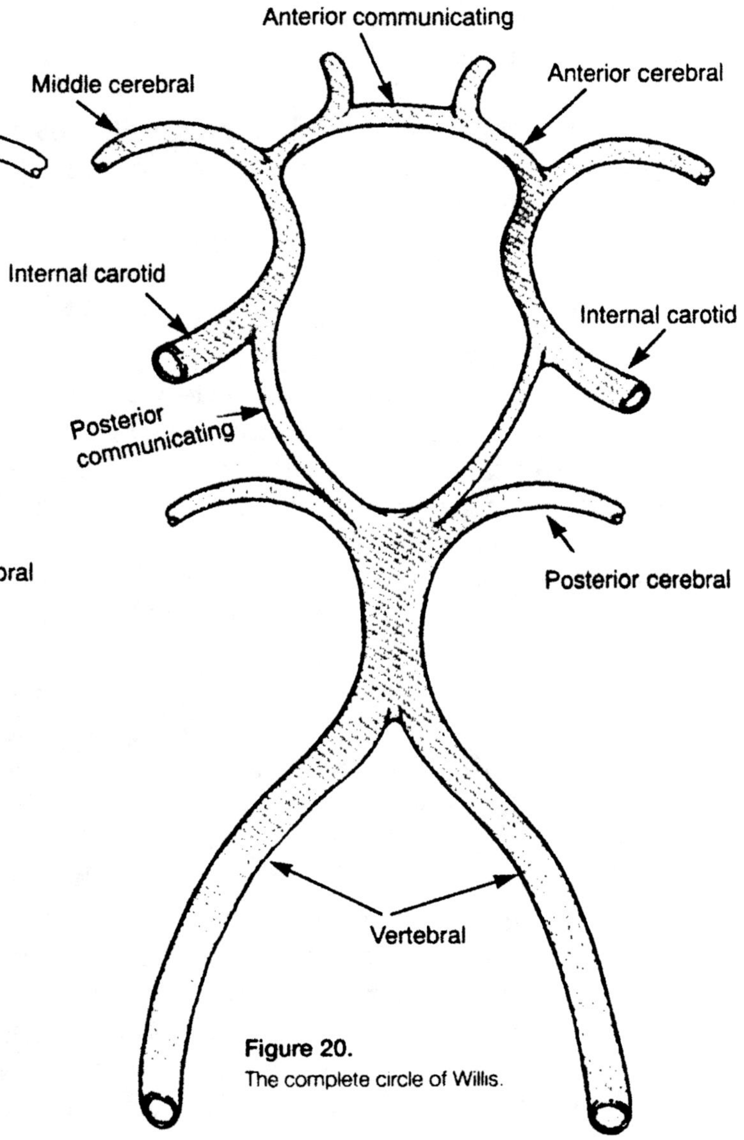

Figure 20.
The complete circle of Willis.

- the right and left posterior cerebral arteries, and
- the right and left posterior communicating arteries.

This posterior half is sometimes called the *vertebrobasilar circulation*, or the vertebrobasilar half of the circle of Willis (Figure 19).

To recap, then, the entire circle of Willis (Figure 20) consists of 14 arteries. The anterior, or carotid, half includes the right and left internal carotid arteries, the right and left anterior cerebral arteries, the right and left middle cerebral arteries, and the single anterior communicating artery. The posterior, or vertebrobasilar, half consists of the right and left vertebral arteries, the single basilar artery, the right and left posterior cerebral arteries, and the right and left posterior communicating arteries.

Diagnostic and Clinical Significance

Besides supplying the brain with oxygenated blood, the circle of Willis serves as a natural connection between the right and left halves of the carotid circulation and between the carotid and vertebrobasilar circulations. These natural side-to-side and posteroanterior connections are extremely important to maintaining blood flow to the brain in the event of serious disease of the carotid arteries.

For instance, if there is significant obstruction of the right internal carotid artery, the left internal carotid can supply blood to the right hemisphere (half) of the brain by sending it across the anterior communicating artery. In other words, the anterior communicating artery would provide a natural side-to-side shunt on its own side of the circle of Willis.

Conversely, the vertebrobasilar arteries could send blood to the right hemisphere by way of the posterior communicating arteries. This would be a back-to-front (posteroanterior) shunt between the two halves of the circle. By the way, an individual vertebral artery cannot be designated as providing the means for this collateral flow, since the right and left vertebral arteries join to form the single basilar artery. Consequently, the system is referred to as vertebrobasilar.

These collateral routes are called *intracranial collaterals*. The possibility for blood flow to detour around obstruction depends on the circle of Willis being intact. In many people, however, the circle of Willis is lacking one or more arteries. As we said earlier, there is often a considerable difference between the way a textbook

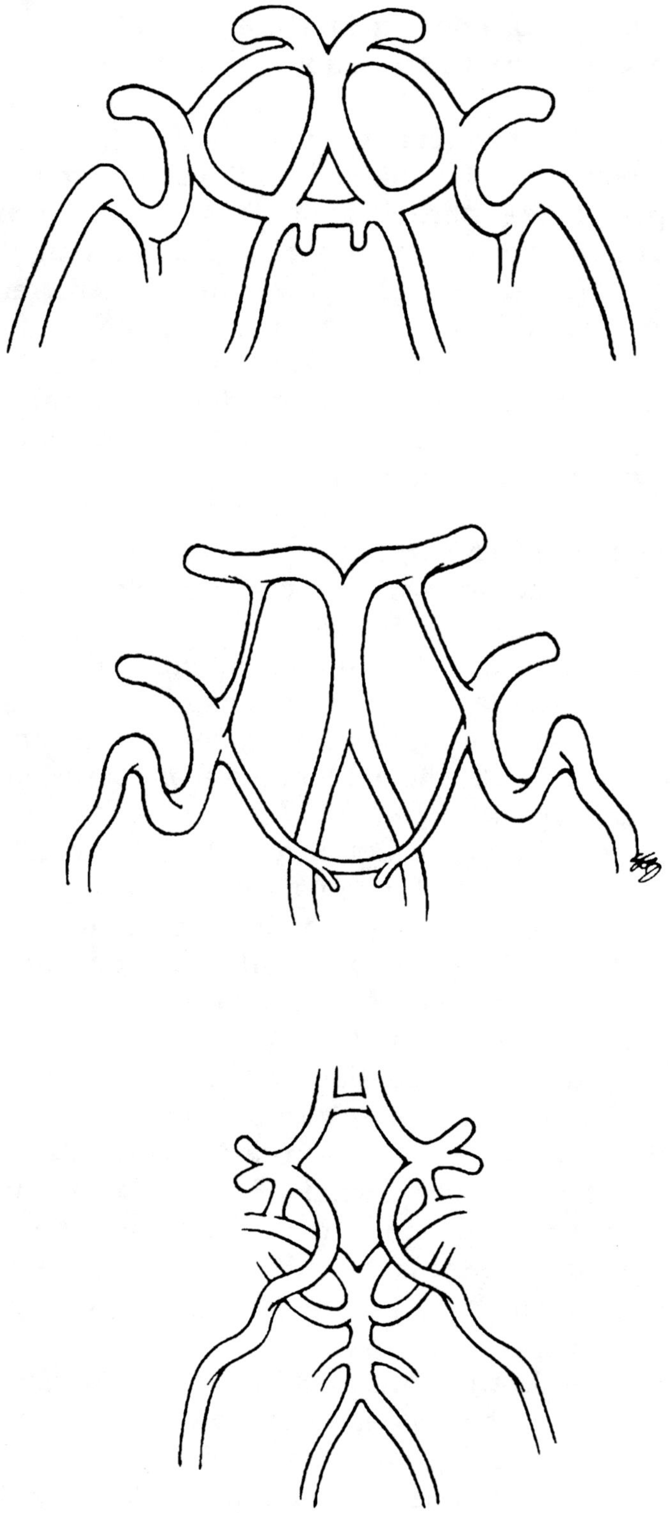

Figure 21.
Three different renderings of the circle of Willis.

says a blood vessel should look and behave and the reality within a human body. This is certainly true of the circle of Willis. Vessels may be missing, or they may begin and/or end in unusual places. The arterial pattern we have described is the one most commonly found and is therefore considered the normal configuration.

In any given individual, the less complete the circle of Willis, the less likely that person is to have natural alternative routes for intracranial blood flow in the event of obstruction. For instance, if the anterior communicating artery is missing, there can be no crossover from the contralateral internal carotid artery. If both posterior communicating arteries are absent, the possibility of a vertebrobasilar supply disappears. And if the anterior communicating artery is missing and even one of the posterior communicating arteries is also missing, there is no possibility of any natural intracranial collateral circulation. The fewer possible collateral routes there are, the more likely it is that the patient will have symptoms—from mild to major—if carotid disease is present.

Learning to Recognize the Intracranial Arteries

As we described it at the outset, the circle of Willis originates in the skull at the base of the brain. But it is not aligned straight up and down, the way, for instance, that the cervical carotid arteries are. Instead, the circle of Willis lies tipped at an angle. This angled position creates a great deal of difficulty for people when it comes to picturing the circle from a drawing on a flat page. (It creates a great deal of difficulty for the medical illustrator, too!)

It is comparatively easy to look at the other arteries of the systemic circulation and picture their course, since looking at the two-dimensional (flat) picture is not that different from looking at a human body. For example, you can look at a drawing of the aorta/iliac artery/femoral artery/popliteal artery progression and identify each vessel. With an angled circular formation, however, it can be quite difficult to identify the individual vessels within the structure.

Figure 21 demonstrates the wide variety of renditions by which the circle of Willis is portrayed. Some medical illustrators attempt to convey the angled nature of the circle by "looking over" the front half toward the rear. Some have you looking "under" the front half toward the vertebrobasilar vessels. Sometimes the artist will "pull up" the front half to try to create a simple up-and-down representation. All these variations can be quite confusing to the person who is trying to recognize the different arteries involved.

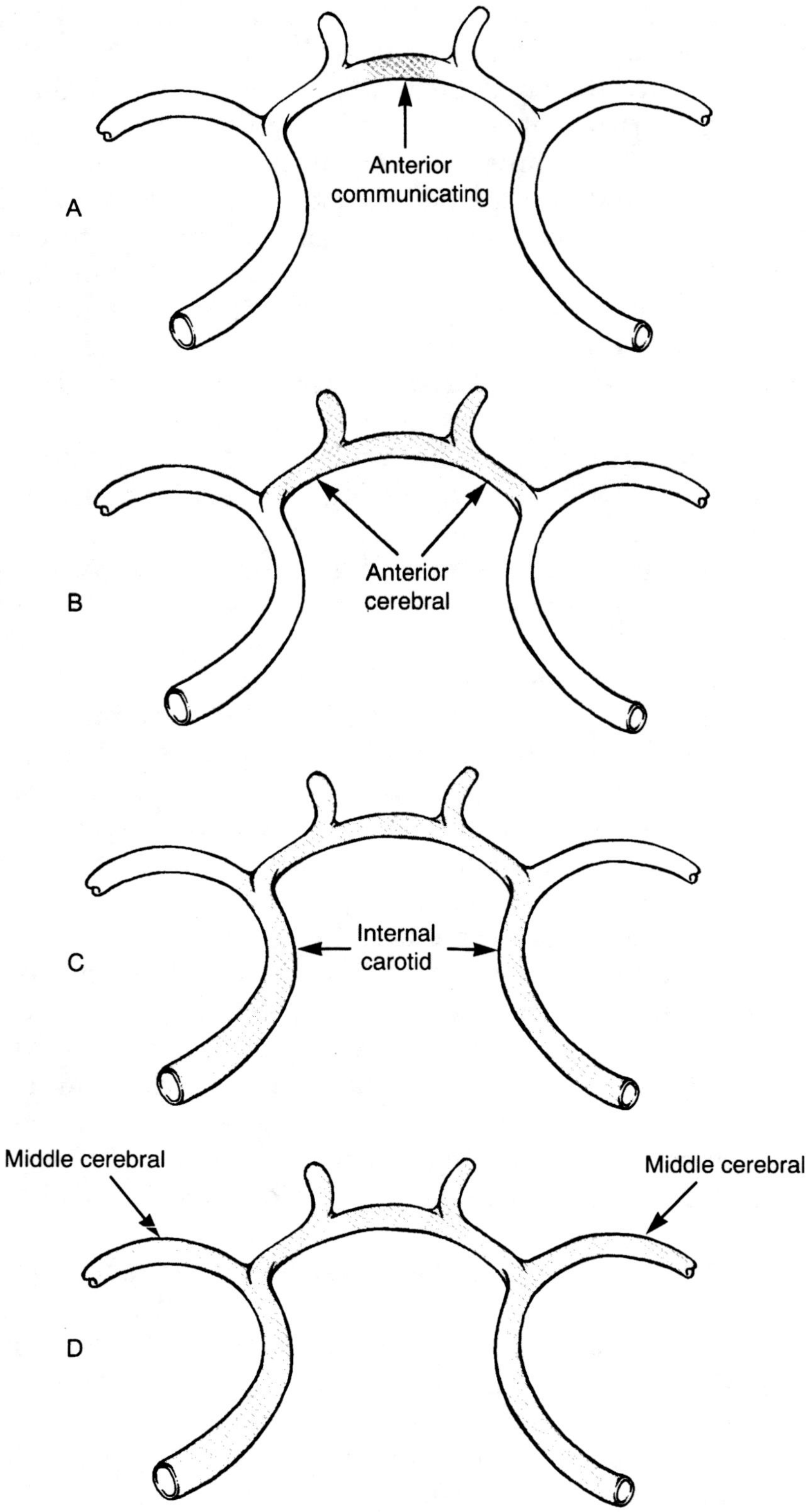

Figure 22A-D.
Identifying the arteries in the anterior half of the circle of Willis.

A difficult task or concept is best learned in simple steps. Toward that end, we have devised a step-by-step process by which you should be able to label each vessel in the circle of Willis no matter how the artist has drawn it. Basically, the method consists of dividing the circle into its two component halves and then looking for landmarks, or clues, that will enable you to begin a systematic identification of one vessel after another.

Your first landmark should be easily recognizable no matter what the artist's rendition is like. In each hemisphere, which single artery will be consistent from one illustration to the next? The words "single artery" are the clue. Both the posterior and the anterior halves of the circle contain seven arteries: three pairs and one single. In each half, the single artery becomes the starting landmark. In the anterior half, this is the anterior communicating artery. In the posterior half, it is the basilar artery. Now, what clues can be used in identifying these single arteries?

Let us begin with the anterior half. In this half of the circle blood can cross over from one side to the other. A structure that allows you to cross from one side to another is a bridge. So, in this half of the circle, you need to look for a bridge. No matter what the drawing looks like otherwise, there will be only one vessel that resembles a bridge, and that vessel will be the anterior communicating artery (Figure 22A).

Now, if you remember that the anterior communicating artery connects the right and left anterior cerebral arteries, you can easily identify those arteries on either side of the bridge (Figure 22B).

Remembering that the anterior cerebral arteries come off the internal carotid artery allows you to find those two vessels (Figure 22C).

Finally, the internal carotid arteries terminate as the middle cerebral arteries, so they must be the remaining vessels (Figure 22D).

Now, probably in less than one minute, you have labeled all the arteries in the anterior half of the circle of Willis. The next step is <u>not</u> to try working your way into the posterior half, but to treat the vertebrobasilar half as a separate entity.

Your first step, as it was with the anterior half, is to find your landmark single artery, in this case the basilar artery. At this point we get a little corny. Remember how pirates are said to mark their maps with an "X" where the treasure was buried? Well, the brain

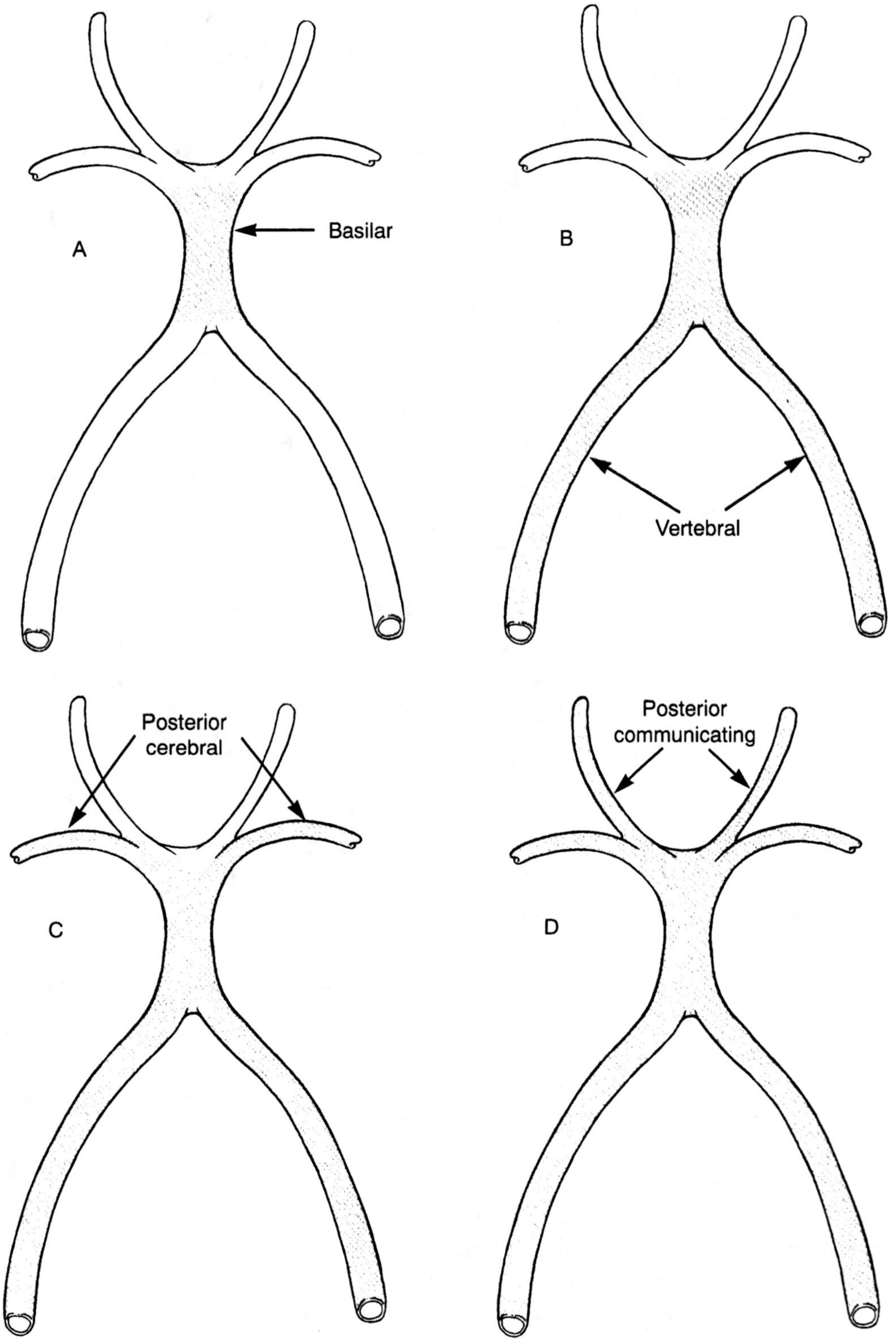

Figure 23A-D.
Identifying the arteries in the posterior half of the circle of Willis.

is a treasure to us: It keeps us alive and functioning. So, as with the pirate map, "X" marks the spot. In all renditions of the posterior half, you should be able to find something that looks like an "X" formation. Sometimes it will be stretched out; sometimes it will look rather short; but it will always resemble the letter "X"—at least slightly. The center of the "X," where its lines cross, is the basilar artery, your starting point (Figure 23A).

You know that the basilar artery is formed by the anastomosis of the right and left vertebral arteries, so the vessels at the base of the "X" are the vertebrals (Figure 23B). The basilar artery bifurcates to form the right and left posterior cerebral arteries, so the upper extensions of the "X" can be identified as those vessels (Figure 23C). Only two arteries remain unlabeled in this half of the circle, so by elimination you know that they must be the right and left posterior communicating arteries (Figure 23D).

Again, in a few seconds, you've named the seven arteries that form half of the circle of Willis, this time the posterior half. Now, by putting the two halves together, you have identified all 14 arteries (Figure 24).

There is one potential pitfall. Many illustrations show several small arteries coming off the basilar artery between the vertebral and posterior cerebral "legs." (That is because in this text we have concentrated on the arteries of the cerebrovascular circulation most important to our concerns.) To avoid confusing these small intracranial arteries with the vertebral and posterior cerebral arteries, make sure you are looking at the very top and very bottom of the "X." In other words, if there are any "legs" below the ones you are considering, those are the vertebral arteries.

You have now traced the carotid and vertebrobasilar circulations from their origins to their intracranial destination. You have also seen how the body can attempt to compensate for carotid disease by using alternative routes in the circle of Willis or in one or more branches of the external carotid artery to supply blood to the brain. Although the patterns we have discussed in this chapter may seem complex, they provide only a general overview of one of the most fascinating areas of the human vasculature.

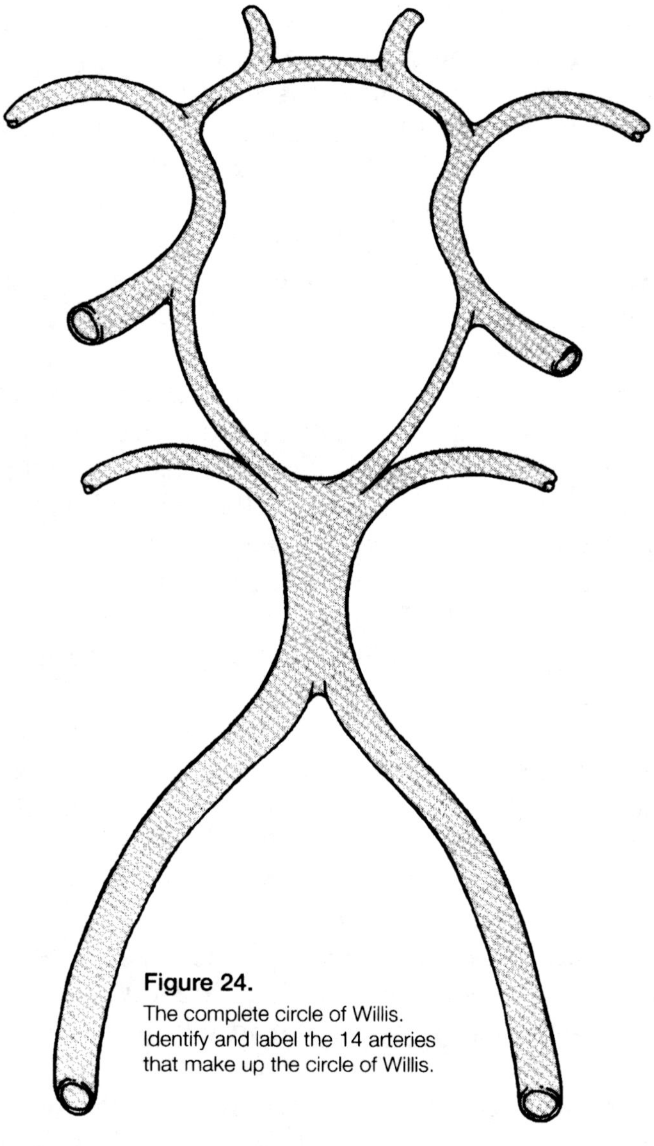

Figure 24.
The complete circle of Willis.
Identify and label the 14 arteries
that make up the circle of Willis.

CHAPTER REVIEW

- The right and left common carotid arteries have different origins. Once formed, however, they follow the same routes.
- The common carotid artery is an exclusively extracranial cerebrovascular artery, and it lies only in the neck, or cervical, region.
- The external carotid artery is also exclusively extracranial.
- The internal carotid artery has both an extracranial cervical portion and an intracranial portion.
- The common carotid artery normally bifurcates at the level of the thyroid cartilage. In this region is also found the carotid bulb, with its sensitive pressoreceptors.
- The major branches of the external carotid artery are the occipital, the facial, the internal maxillary (which terminates as the infraorbital), and the superficial temporal arteries.
- The major branches of the internal carotid artery are the ophthalmic, the anterior cerebral, and the middle cerebral arteries.
- The three major branches of the ophthalmic artery are the supraorbital, the frontal, and the nasal arteries.
- The seven vessels of the anterior, or carotid, circulation are the right and left internal carotid, the right and left anterior cerebral, the right and left middle cerebral, and the anterior communicating arteries.
- The seven vessels of the posterior, or vertebrobasilar, circulation are the right and left vertebral, the basilar, the right and left posterior cerebral, and the right and left posterior communicating arteries.
- The seven vessels of the anterior, or carotid, circulation together with the seven vessels of the posterior, or vertebrobasilar, circulation join to form the circle of Willis.

CHAPTER

7

The Systemic Circulation: The Peripheral Veins

Learning the anatomy of the venous system should be relatively easy at this point, since just about one-third of it shares names and locations with the arteries you have already learned. Nevertheless, there are some exceptions. Also, when we talked about the peripheral arteries, we spoke only of the arterial system. The arterioles and the arterial capillaries were not discussed as a system and were given no specific names. In discussing the venous portion of the peripheral systemic circulation, however, we will deal with three different groups, or systems: the deep veins, the superficial veins, and the perforating or communicating veins.

Another difference is that in tracing the course of the arteries, which move blood away from the heart, we spoke of vessels branching or dividing, getting smaller as they traveled from the heart to the periphery. The veins, in contrast, are the "back half" of the closed-loop circulatory pattern we described in Section I. Blood

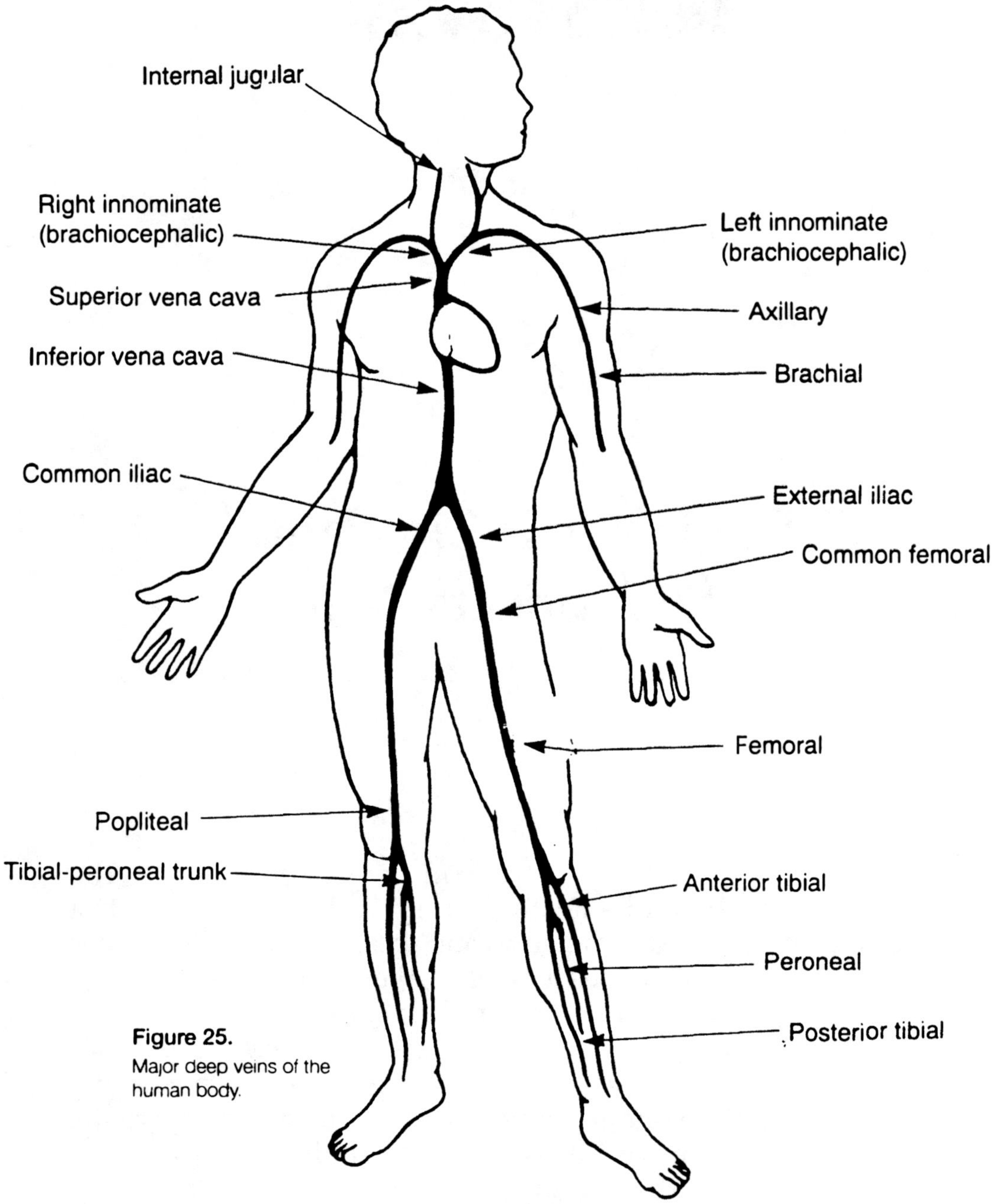

Figure 25.
Major deep veins of the human body.

flows through the veins toward the heart, and that is how we will trace the course of each system of the venous circulation: starting with the periphery and working back toward the heart. As veins join with other veins, they get bigger, not smaller. With that understanding, we will begin with the deep veins (Figure 25).

THE DEEP VEINS

The *deep veins* are called that because of where they are in relation to skin and muscle. All veins lie under the skin, but some veins are more deeply situated than others. If you were to peel back the skin from a leg, you would find a semitransparent, whitish membrane holding the muscles together. This membrane, which looks like the covering on a leg of lamb at the supermarket, is made up of fibrous tissue and is called the *fascia*. The deep veins are those that lie under both skin and fascia.

In the extremities, deep veins are surrounded by muscle, a fact that is important to the flow of venous blood. (That relationship is discussed in Section V, Venous Hemodynamics.) The deep veins of the body lie next to the major arteries and almost always share their names. There are some exceptions to the arterial/deep venous similarity, and three of them occur more or less as a group in the upper half of the body. For this reason we will start with the deep veins of the upper extremity.

Deep Veins Originating in the Upper Extremities

Blood returning from the digital (finger) veins empties into a venous network in the hand called the *palmar* or *volar arch*. Just as in the arterial system, there is both a deep and a superficial arch in the hand, and these unite to form the beginning of the *radial* and *ulnar veins* of the forearm. Not all anatomists agree that these veins, which share the name and location of the radial and ulnar arteries, are truly deep veins. They have somewhat superficial sections as well as deep sections, and consequently some texts list them as deep veins and some do not.

The radial and ulnar veins move proximally in the forearm, next to the arteries, and they join in the area of the antecubital fossa to form the *brachial vein*. The brachial vein has no superficial component, and therefore some anatomists consider it to be the first of the true deep veins of the upper extremity. It runs through the arm beside the brachial artery, gradually increasing in size as it goes along.

As the brachial vein enters the axilla (armpit), it takes on the name of its new location and becomes the *axillary vein.* As it emerges from the axilla and passes under the clavicle, it is called the *subclavian vein.* It is then joined by the *vertebral vein,* which has passed through the same transverse processes of the cervical vertebrae as the subclavian artery (only carrying blood in the opposite direction). The joined subclavian and vertebral vein then travel to the first of the artery/deep venous exceptions.

There is only one innominate (brachiocephalic) artery, but there are two *innominate/brachiocephalic veins.* The innominate artery bifurcates to form the right subclavian artery and the right common carotid artery. The innominate vein is formed by the joining of the subclavian vein and the second of our exceptions, the internal jugular vein.

In the arterial circulation, there is a vessel on each side of the neck called the common carotid artery. In the deep venous circulation there is no "carotid vein" to correspond with that artery. Instead, the right and left *internal jugular veins* run alongside the carotid arteries. So, on the right side, the right subclavian vein joins the right internal jugular vein to form the *right innominate vein.* On the left side, where there is no equivalent innominate artery, the left subclavian vein and the left internal jugular vein form the *left innominate vein.* The right and left innominate veins anastomose to form the third of the arterial/deep venous exceptions: the superior vena cava.

The two *venae cavae* are the venous equivalent of the aorta. Just as all blood supplied by the arterial system comes from the heart by way of the aorta, all blood drained by the venous system returns to the heart by way of one of the venae cavae. The *superior vena cava,* which is formed by the anastomosis of the innominate veins, is the larger of the two. The inferior vena cava, which drains the abdomen, is discussed later. The superior vena cava is so named because it receives the venous return from the upper portion of the body (head, neck, thorax, and upper extremities) and is situated above (superior to) the heart. The plural form <u>venae cavae</u> is generally used in speaking of the superior and inferior vena cava together.

Deep Veins Originating in the Lower Extremities

To find the last arterial/deep venous exception it is necessary to go to the distal lower extremity. In the foot, a situation exists similar

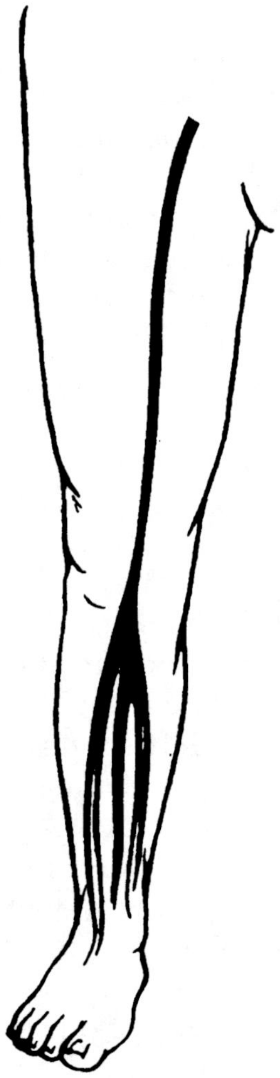

Figure 26.
Paired deep venous branches in the calf—one example of multiple deep veins in the leg.

to that in the hand: Both a deep and a superficial arch structure receive venous drainage from the digits (toes). Beginning at the ankle, we find the first of the exclusively deep veins. Just as in the arterial circulation, the leg contains *anterior tibial, posterior tibial,* and *peroneal* vessels. But the arterial system has one of each, whereas the venous system has several of each (Figure 26). Two, occasionally three, or, more rarely, four anterior tibial, posterior tibial, and peroneal veins may be found in the leg in normal individuals. This multiplicity of named deep veins in the leg contributes to the difficulty of assessing small deep venous thromboses (clots) in this area. These paired (or tripled, or quadrupled) veins move proximally along the leg next to the arteries whose names they share.

The joining of the leg veins is similar to the division of the infrapopliteal arteries. The popliteal artery first divides to form the anterior tibial artery and the tibial-peroneal trunk, which then divides to become the posterior tibial and peroneal arteries. In the venous system, the *posterior tibial* and *peroneal veins* come together first and are then joined by the *anterior tibial vein.* All these veins, joined together, form the *popliteal vein.*

Before going on, we should review the arterial/ deep venous exceptions. Two are exceptions in name and two in number. The two "name" exceptions are the internal jugular vein/ common carotid artery equivalents and the venae cavae/ aorta equivalents. The "number" exceptions are one innominate artery versus two innominate veins and one infrapopliteal artery on each side versus two (or more) infrapopliteal veins.

Near the popliteal fossa, the infrapopliteal veins join to become the *popliteal vein.* This vein leaves the fossa and enters the thigh as the *femoral* (formerly "superficial femoral") *vein.* The femoral vein is a deep vein; it runs through the adductor canal along the medial side of the superficial femoral artery. As the femoral vein moves proximally, it joins the *profunda* or *deep femoral vein* and enters the region of the inguinal ligament. There it becomes the *common femoral vein.* The femoral vein and common femoral vein always are situated medial to the superficial and common femoral arteries.

Moving proximally to the level of the ilium (the hip bone), the common femoral vein becomes the *external iliac vein.* It then joins the *internal iliac,* or *hypogastric,* vein to become the *common iliac vein.* Finally, at the level of the umbilicus, the right and left

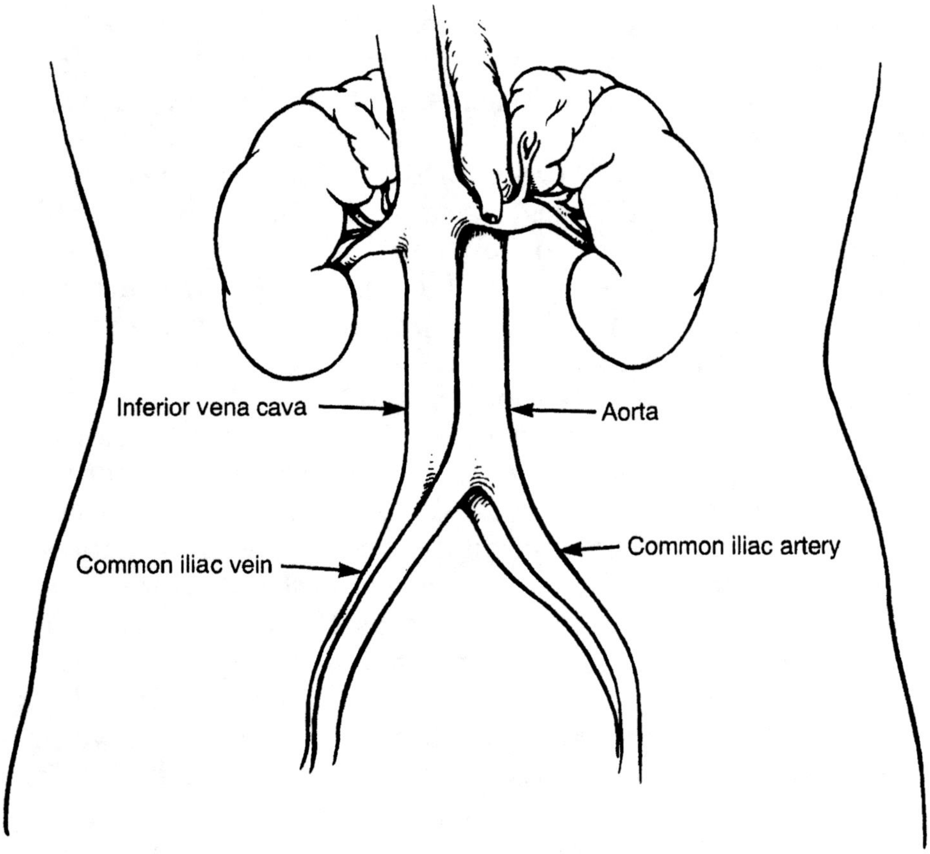

Figure 27.
Coexistence of major vessels in the limited space of the abdominal cavity.

common iliac veins anastomose to form the beginning of the *inferior vena cava.*

The inferior vena cava and the abdominal aorta are paired vessels, both of which arise from paired vessels at their distal margin. However, there is only so much room in which these six major vessels can exist. Look at Figure 27, and you will see how the body allows these veins and arteries to fit into the available space. The right common iliac artery actually lies atop the left common iliac vein so that the inferior vena cava and the aorta can lie side by side. This position sometimes causes compression of the left common iliac vein and may occasionally be a factor in certain noninvasive tests of the lower extremity.

The inferior vena cava moves proximally through the abdomen, gathering return blood from different visceral and pelvic veins. As it reaches the level of the heart, it joins with the superior vena cava to empty all the returning venous blood into the right atrium, where it begins the circulatory cycle all over again.

THE SUPERFICIAL VEINS

The *superficial veins* are those that are located under the skin but above the fascia. These are the veins that can actually be seen beneath the skin, especially if they become distended as varicose veins.

For those of you interested in trivia: The superficial veins are the reason nobility and royalty came to be called "blue-blooded." Until fairly recent times, suntans were shunned by anyone with money; the richer you were, the more likely you were to avoid sun exposure altogether. Wealthy women and noble ladies used to shield their skin from the sun and even bathe in milk to keep their complexions as pale as possible. A tanned complexion was a sign of being poor; peasants who had to labor in the sun all day developed darker, "tougher" skin. In old pictures of cowboys, their skin looks as leathery as their saddles.

The superficial veins of the body carry unoxygenated blood, which is darker than arterial blood and looks bluish under the skin. With very pale skin the blue tint is very obvious. So, wealthy aristocrats who could afford to shun the sun had visible blue veins, unlike the suntanned peasants/slaves/serfs. Hence, the nobility came to be called "blue bloods." Now, back to anatomy.

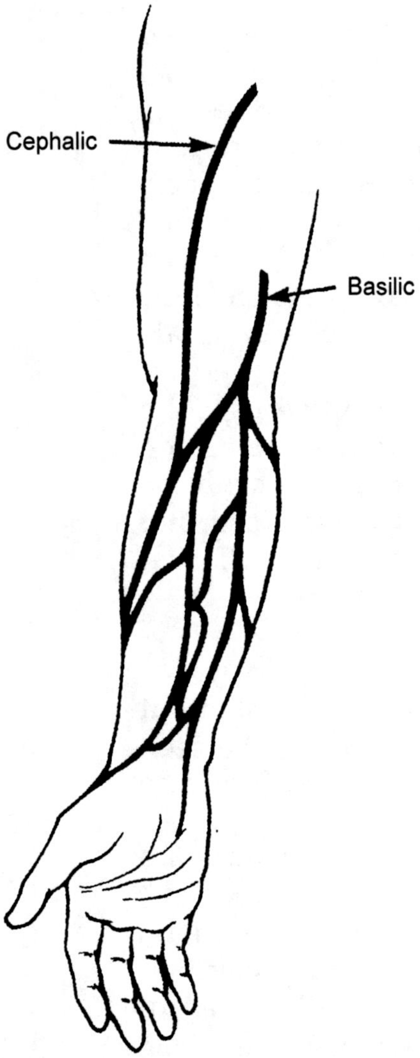

Figure 28.
Superficial veins of the upper extremity.

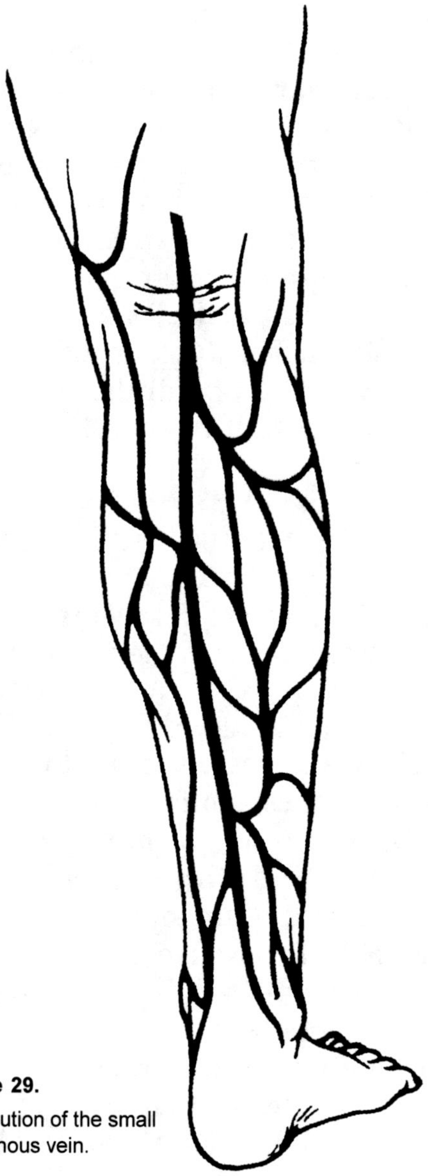

Figure 29.
Distribution of the small saphenous vein.

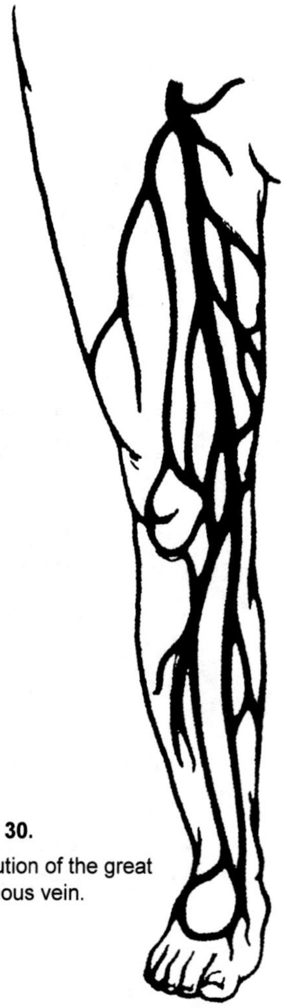

Figure 30.
Distribution of the great saphenous vein.

Superficial Veins of the Upper Extremities

In the hand, as already mentioned, there are superficial as well as deep venous structures called palmar, or volar, arches. In the forearm, the superficial veins form a complex network spreading out over the circumference of the limb. Then, in the arm, these forearm veins join to form two larger superficial veins.

The superficial veins running along the lateral aspect of the arm are called the *cephalic veins,* while those on the medial aspect are called the *basilic veins* (Figure 28). The pattern of distribution for these superficial veins of the upper extremity is different for each person, and it even differs from one side to the other in the same individual. The cephalic and basilic veins empty into the deep venous system via the axillary vein.

Superficial Veins of the Lower Extremities

The lower extremity also has two sets of superficial veins. Starting posterior to the lateral malleolus and running along the posterior aspect of the leg are the veins that form the *small saphenous network* (Figure 29). The posterolateral and posteromedial branches of the small saphenous vein join, then move deep into the interior of the leg by perforating the fascia in the upper third of the calf. The small saphenous network empties into the popliteal vein, usually at the middle portion of the popliteal fossa.

Beginning, again, at the dorsum of the foot, but this time anterior to the medial malleolus, is the *great saphenous vein.* This superficial vein is an extremely important one, especially in surgery, where it is used as material for bypass grafts. Its branches, or tributaries, extend over the anterior, medial, and lateral aspects of the limb, but the route of its main trunk is reasonably well defined (Figure 30). After its origin in the foot, the great saphenous vein passes superiorly along the medial aspect of the leg. In the area of the knee it swings toward the back of the limb. To picture this shift in direction, we need to talk briefly about bones.

The long bone of the thigh is the femur. The distal end of the femur is located at the knee joint. By looking at this joint on your own limb, you can easily see and palpate two large, rounded bony projections, or bulges, one on either side of the joint above the patella (kneecap). These two projections are called the *lateral* and the *medial condyle of the femur.* When the great saphenous vein shifts direction, it swings behind the medial condyle of the femur

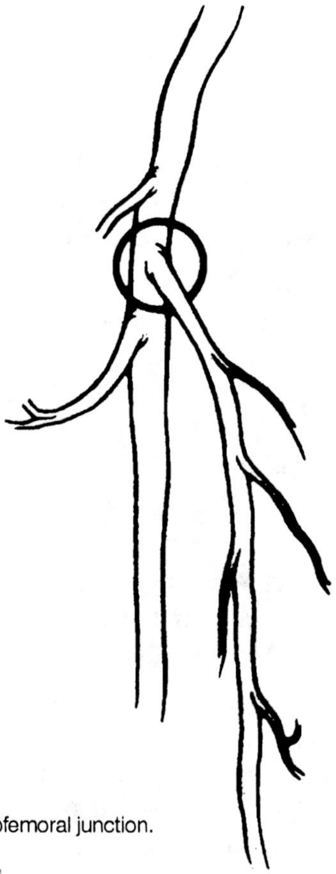

Figure 31.
The saphenofemoral junction.

into the thigh. It remains in the posteromedial aspect of the thigh as it continues upward toward its ultimate anastomosis with the deep venous system.

The great saphenous network connects with the deep venous system a few centimeters below the inguinal ligament. Like the small saphenous network it must penetrate the fascia to reach the deep veins. The juncture of the cephalad end of the great saphenous system with the deep venous system is called the *saphenofemoral junction* (Figure 31).

This junction is an important location in diagnosing pathologic conditions. A thrombus (clot) in the great saphenous system may propagate (extend or move) into the deep venous system by means of the saphenofemoral junction. Such a thrombus would be entering the deep venous system at the level of the common femoral vein, meaning that it would obstruct a vein that receives blood from most of the lower extremity. This creates a condition that is potentially very serious.

In addition to their respective depths, the deep and superficial veins differ in another way, especially in the lower limbs. The walls of the saphenous veins are somewhat stronger than those of the deep leg veins. This makes sense when you consider their relative positions. The deep veins are buried within the muscle masses of the lower limbs, under the fascial layer, and they are supported by these structures. The superficial veins have only a thin covering of skin for protection and support. However, the strength of the saphenous veins is limited; they cannot carry large amounts of blood at any one time. This creates a potential problem.

The veins of the legs have a special burden; they must carry blood back to the heart against the force of gravity. How they accomplish this task is discussed in Section V. But without knowing anything about hemodynamics (the study of blood flow), you can see that if the only juncture with the deep venous system were at the back of the knee and in the groin, the saphenous sytem would be continually burdened with a large amount of blood. This is avoided by the body's system for steadily siphoning off, or draining, the returning blood on its way to the saphenofemoral and saphenopopliteal junctions. That system forms the third portion of the venous circulation.

THE PERFORATING (COMMUNICATING) VEINS

The *perforating* or *communicating veins* allow blood in the superficial veins to remain at manageable levels. Different texts favor one or the other of these names, but either is correct. These veins penetrate the fascia, hence the name perforating. They also allow direct flow of blood between the deep and superficial veins, hence the name communicating. Communicating veins are found in the foot, leg, and thigh, but they are most extensive in the leg.

Recall that veins have bicuspid semilunar valves along their length. The distribution of these valves varies somewhat from person to person, but they are present in deep, superficial, and perforating/communicating veins. In the deep and superficial veins, the valves are oriented to direct the movement of blood back toward the heart. The valves in the perforating/ communicating veins, however, direct the flow from the superficial veins toward the deep veins. Although the number and distribution of the venous valves varies among individuals, there are some general guidelines regarding their occurrence.

In the leg, some veins have fewer valves than others. Among the deep veins, posterior tibial veins usually contain from nine to nineteen valves, the anterior tibials from nine to eleven, and the peroneal veins only about seven. The femoral vein generally has three valves, with one usually situated proximally within one centimeter of the inguinal ligament. About one person in four has a valve in the external iliac vein, but valves in the common iliac vein are extremely rare. Superficial veins usually have far fewer valves than deep veins. For instance, the great and small saphenous veins combined generally have only about seven to nine valves.

We have now discussed the deep, superficial, and perforating/communicating veins of the trunk and extremities, and we have identified the internal jugular vein as being paired with the carotid artery. But we have not named any intracranial veins. That is because there are no veins, as such, in the cranial cavity. The large spaces within the cranium that contain venous blood are called *sinuses.* (These should not be confused with the air-filled cavities in the bones of the skull that are also called sinuses.) These cranial sinuses are simply large channels which form an anastomosing network between the layers of dura mater

of the brain (the outermost and toughest of the three membranes or meninges that cover the brain and the spinal cord). They receive the venous drainage from the brain and empty it into the veins of the scalp or those at the base of the skull. In fact, two of these sinuses, the right and left transverse (lateral) sinuses, actually become the right and left internal jugular veins.

CHAPTER REVIEW

- The peripheral venous circulation may be divided into three systems: the deep veins, the superficial veins, and the perforating, or communicating, veins.
- The deep veins lie under the skin and the fascia; the superficial veins lie under the skin but above the fascia.
- The perforating/communicating veins provide a connection between the deep and superficial veins.
- The deep veins of the body lie next to the major arteries and usually share a common name. The exceptions are the internal jugular vein/common carotid artery pair and the superior and inferior venae cavae/aorta pair.
- Two other exceptions to the deep vein/artery similarity involve number rather than name. There are two innominate/brachiocephalic veins, but there is only one innominate/brachiocephalic artery. There is only one each of the infrapopliteal arteries (anterior tibial, posterior tibial, and peroneal), but there are two (or more) of each of the infrapopliteal veins.
- The superficial veins of the upper extremity are the cephalic and basilic veins; those of the lower extremity are the great and small saphenous veins.
- The great saphenous vein empties into the deep system via the saphenofemoral junction; the small saphenous vein empties via the saphenopopliteal junction.
- The perforating/communicating veins allow blood from the superficial veins to be continuously siphoned into the deep system to prevent excessive volume in the superficial veins.

SECTION FOUR

Arterial Hemodynamics

Understanding the nature and location of the blood vessels, that is, their anatomy, provides only a partial picture of the circulatory system. It is also important to understand how and why blood moves, or fails to move, through these different channels. In other words, we now need to look at vascular physiology, and especially that part of it known as hemodynamics.

Physiology is the study of how a living organism, or a portion of a living organism, functions. Thus, *vascular physiology* is the study of how the parts of the vascular anatomy that you have just learned about function. *Dynamics* is the study of an organism or a system in motion; thus, *hemodynamics* is the science concerned with the movement of blood through the circulatory system.

To make vascular physiology easier to learn, we have divided the information into arterial and venous aspects.

CHAPTER

8

Characteristics of Arterial Blood Flow

One concept about arterial blood flow is familiar to just about everyone: We know that blood moves through our bodies because of the pushing, or pumping, action of the heart. Since the arteries are the vessels that carry blood away from the heart, it stands to reason that they would be the vessels most directly affected by the heart's pumping. And that is true. For the most part, the pumping of the heart—its pulsation—is a major factor in arterial, but not in venous, physiology. Of course, the arterial and venous vessels are all part of a closed-loop system. Consequently, what affects one part of the system has some bearing on the other part. However, pulsatile influence on the venous system is generally minimal, as you will see in Section V.

THE PHASES OF ARTERIAL PULSATION

Because the heart beats, or pulsates, to force blood out of its chambers and into the arterial system, the blood in the arteries is said to be *pulsatile*. This pulsatile nature of arterial blood flow is

the first concept to be learned about arterial hemodynamics. The pulsation of the heart occurs in two phases, systole and diastole. These two phases of the cardiac cycle were first identified and named by Galen, the Roman physician credited with being the first to discover that blood circulates (see Section II).

Systole is the Greek word for "shorten." Muscles contract by shortening and tightening; therefore the first portion of the cardiac cycle, when the heart muscle is contracting, is called *systole.* If we speak of the *atrial systole,* we are speaking only of the contraction of the atria, which forces blood into the ventricles. *Ventricular systole* refers to the contraction of the ventricles, which forces blood out through the pulmonary artery and the ascending thoracic aorta. Generally, when the term systole is used alone, it means the contraction of the ventricles.

The word *diastole* comes from the Greek word that means "to dilate," but actually refers to the resting half of the cardiac cycle. Muscles cannot contract continuously; they have to relax intermittently in order to function. So, between each systolic phase and the next, a diastolic phase occurs as part of the cardiac cycle, or heartbeat. During diastole, the heart is not contracting. It can therefore fill up with the blood it needs for the next period of contraction. As blood fills the chambers of the heart, it actually does become somewhat larger, or dilated. For this reason, diastole is often called the dilatation phase, rather than the relaxation phase, of the cardiac cycle, and in this sense the Greek word of origin is correct.

BLOOD PRESSURE

When you measure blood pressure with a sphygmomanometer and stethoscope, you take two readings, expressed in numbers such as 120/80. The higher number is the systolic pressure, and the lower number is the diastolic pressure. *Systolic pressure* represents the force that the blood is exerting against the arterial wall as the heart contracts. Arterial pressure is always at its highest during systole. *Diastolic pressure* represents the force exerted during maximum relaxation of the heart muscle; it is the lowest pressure recorded during the cardiac cycle. Even though arterial pressure varies over the cardiac cycle, it is always higher than the pressure in the normal venous system.

Changes in blood pressure within different vessels, and at different times, account for part of the reason that blood moves where and how it does within the body. We will talk more about the influence of pressure on blood movement in Chapter 10.

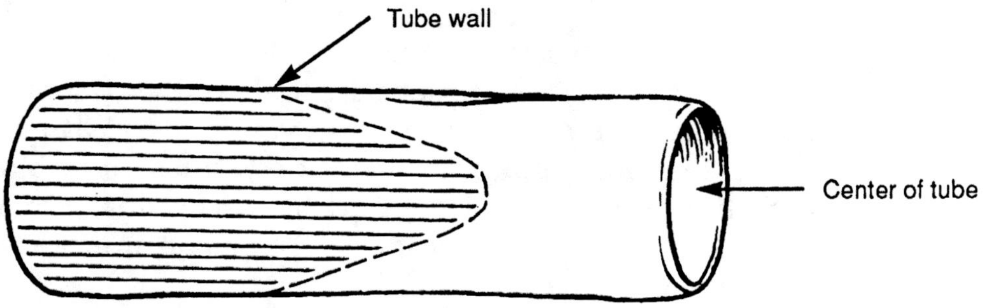

Figure 32.
Laminar arterial flow in a parabolic flow profile.

Now you know that arterial blood pulsates because of the beating of the heart. You also know that pressure within the artery varies from one phase of the cardiac cycle to the next. Now, what about some of the other characteristics of arterial flow?

LAMINAR FLOW

Besides being pulsatile, arterial blood flow has another characteristic important to noninvasive testing. That characteristic is related to the manner in which blood cells are distributed as they move through the artery. Normally, blood is arranged in a layered fashion within the arterial *lumen*, or channel. The adjective "laminar" means "arranged in layers," so we say that normal arterial blood flow is *laminar flow*. In laminar flow, the blood cells in the layer closest to the arterial wall travel at the slowest velocity. (*Velocity* means speed plus direction.) In fact, blood cells in the outer layers move so slowly they are virtually standing still, or static. The cells in the middle of the lumen, the "center stream," move the fastest.

Suppose you could take a section of artery filled with blood and remove it from the body with all its blood layers undisturbed. Now suppose further that you could take those layers and peel them off, one by one, coloring each layer so that you could distinguish one from another and identify its proper position in the "stack." Finally, you place those color-coded layers at one end of the now empty artery and hold a race. You line all the cells up in their appropriate layers and let each layer move at its normal speed, then take a "freeze frame" photograph of the action before the fastest layer has gone all the way through.

You would find that the cells in the middle layer had traveled farthest, while those along the walls had gone the shortest distance. The layers in between would be arranged in graduated curves. If you then draw a line along the edges of these layers, you will have a geometric shape called a parabola (Figure 32). You have just demonstrated to yourself why laminar arterial flow can be described as having a *parabolic flow profile*, another concept important to vascular diagnostic techniques.

THE PARABOLIC FLOW PROFILE

In reality, the parabolic flow profile best describes what happens to fluid flowing in steady, nonpulsatile fashion through a vessel that has straight, rigid walls. This is a situation quite different from the pulsatile flow of blood through flexible arteries that curve and

twist through the body. Even so, an approximation of true parabolic flow does occur in certain arteries at certain times within the cardiac cycle. During systole, the flow profile in the smaller arteries does become almost truly parabolic. As the size of the artery increases, this parabolic profile is less and less likely to occur. In fact, the profile of flow through the largest artery, the aorta, is actually more blunted than parabolic in shape.

We have already said that variations in intraarterial pressure occur during different phases of the cardiac cycle. In addition, differences in flow profiles are generated within specific arteries during the course of any given heartbeat. During diastole, the speed of blood slows somewhat compared with systole. Consequently, the flow profile becomes increasingly blunted. This means that even in arteries that generate an approximately parabolic flow profile, that parabolic shape exists only at maximum systole. However, when blood flow is turbulent, as it may be in a *stenosed* (obstructed) vessel, the flow profile is blunted throughout the cardiac cycle. Can you see the diagnostic significance of this fact?

Now you know that arterial blood flow is pulsatile, that blood cells are arranged in the arteries in laminar fashion, and that arterial blood flow is said to generate a parabolic flow profile. But why? To understand what causes blood to move into or out of a specific vessel at a given velocity, it is necessary to understand something about energy, pressure, and resistance. All these factors work together in circulating blood through the body.

CHAPTER REVIEW

- Arterial blood flow is pulsatile because of the pumping action of the heart. Pulsation has two phases, systole and diastole.
- Systole is the contracting, or pumping, phase of the heart cycle; diastole is the resting, or relaxation, phase.
- Normal arterial flow moves in laminar (layered) fashion within the vessel lumen. In laminar flow, the cells at midstream move the fastest; those along the vessel wall move the slowest.
- Laminar flow produces a characteristic blood flow profile—called a parabolic flow profile—in certain arteries during systole.

CHAPTER

9

Energy Concepts

Energy has many definitions. In the science of physics, energy is defined as the capacity for doing work (which also has a special meaning in physics) and for overcoming resistance. It is that definition of energy we will be talking about in this chapter as it relates to the movement of blood within the body. But even within that definition, energy takes a number of different forms. The concepts of energy important to hemodynamics are kinetic energy, potential energy, and fluid energy.

KINETIC ENERGY

Kinetic energy is the energy of something in motion. The aspect of kinetic energy we are concerned with relates to the movement of fluids, specifically blood, within a vessel. Kinetic energy is related to another concept in physics, inertia.

Inertia is the tendency of objects (called "bodies" in physics) to maintain their status quo. If an object is at rest, whether it is a

blood clot lying within a vessel, a rock lying on a mountainside, or yourself on the couch watching TV, the concept of inertia explains that body's tendency to remain at rest. If something is already moving, for example, a car at 55 mph entering a curve, inertia explains its tendency to continue moving in the direction in which it was going rather than to alter its course.

To determine how much kinetic energy is present, you need to look at two factors, its mass and its velocity. *Mass*, for the purposes of our discussion, can be simply defined as the accumulation of molecules that stick together, or adhere, to form the object. *Velocity* is speed plus direction. The kinetic energy of, for example, a given collection of blood cells is equal to one-half its mass multiplied by its velocity squared, or:

$$K = \frac{M}{2} V^2$$

K = kinetic energy
M = mass
V = velocity

Study this formula more closely, and you see that the velocity of an object has a greater impact on its kinetic energy than its mass does. After all, in determining K by this equation, you are <u>dividing</u> the mass by 2 but <u>squaring</u> the velocity. Inertia, like velocity, does not change the mass (the density of the blood, for example) but does slow it down. Inertial loss is reflected as a decrease in the velocity of flow.

POTENTIAL ENERGY

Potential energy is the opposite of kinetic energy: It is the energy of something at rest rather than in motion. Visualize a jack-in-the-box. The clown head on the toy is mounted on a spring. With the box closed, this spring is tightly coiled, ready to pop up. That is potential energy. When a child opens the box, the coiled spring opens and the toy pops out. The spring's uncoiling represents kinetic energy.

In hemodynamics, potential energy is a combination of intravascular pressure and gravitational potential energy. *Intravascular pressure* is produced by a combination of the muscular contraction of the heart, the hydrostatic pressure exerted by the blood, and the static filling pressure of the blood. (Other factors

such as friction also enter in, but we are trying to keep this explanation as simple as possible so that you can learn the most basic of the principles involved.)

Hydrostatic pressure can most simply be defined as the pressure exerted by a fluid within a closed system: oil in a pipeline or blood in the circulatory system. Hydrostatic pressure is discussed more fully in the section on venous hemodynamics, since it has a greater influence on venous than on arterial blood flow. The equation for determining hydrostatic pressure reflects the three factors that determine it:

$$HP = -\rho g h$$

HP = hydrostatic pressure
ρ = specific gravity
g = acceleration due to gravity
h = height above a specified reference point

The specific gravity of an object, in this case blood, is its weight compared to a given standard. Acceleration due to gravity is the rate at which something speeds up as it falls because of the effect of gravity. The height above a specified reference point, in this case, would be the height above the right atrium of the heart. This distance is always expressed in centimeters (cm).

The *static filling pressure* of the blood is the pressure that exists because of the relationship between the amount of blood in a vessel and the elasticity of the vessel walls. This pressure is unrelated to the movement of the blood within the vessel.

Again, the contraction of the heart, the hydrostatic pressure, and the static filling pressure, interrelated with gravitational potential energy, give us the potential energy of the blood flow. *Gravitational potential energy* represents the capacity of a quantity of blood to do work, based on its position above a specified reference point. The higher an object is above any given point, the greater the effect gravity has on it. (You probably have heard examples of this, such as the capacity of a penny dropped from the top of the Empire State Building to badly dent the roof of a car parked below.)

The formula for determining gravitational potential energy should look familiar. It is:

$$GPE = +\rho g h$$

GPH = gravitational potential energy
ρ = specific gravity
g = acceleration due to gravity
h = height above a specified reference point

You should have recognized that this equation is almost identical to the one for hydrostatic pressure. The only difference between the right side of these two equations is the sign used with the ρ. In determining hydrostatic pressure, you use the negative value of the specific gravity, acceleration, and height. To calculate gravitational potential energy, you use the positive value of these factors. In other words, these factors frequently cancel each other out. To finally arrive at the potential energy, you combine (add) gravitational potential energy and intravascular pressure.

FLUID ENERGY

The last of the kinds of energy important to hemodynamics is *fluid energy*, which is the total, or combination, of kinetic and potential energy present. In the form of an equation:

$$FE = KE + PE$$

FE = fluid energy
KE = kinetic energy
PE = potential energy

In other words, once you know the kinetic energy and the potential energy, simple addition will give you the fluid energy.

VISCOSITY

Besides inertia, another factor we have not yet discussed contributes to loss of energy. That factor is the *viscosity*, or stickiness, of the blood. The adjective form is viscous. These words derive from the Latin word for birdlime, a sticky substance made by boiling mistletoe berries or holly bark and smeared over twigs and branches to catch birds. A viscous fluid is sticky; that is, its molecules tend to stick to one another so that it is semifluid or gelatinous rather than thin and watery. A very thick, or viscous, fluid is said to have a high degree of viscosity.

What does viscosity have to do with energy loss? The stronger the attraction between its molecules, the more difficult it is for a substance to flow. In other words, a substance with a high degree

of viscosity has a high resistance to flowing. (There is more about resistance in Chapter 10.) For instance, mineral oil has a higher viscosity than water. If you tip over a glass of water, the water will run out quickly. If you tip over a glass containing an equal amount of mineral oil, the oil will move out much more slowly. So, in addition to inertial losses of energy in blood flow, energy losses due to viscosity can occur.

Two factors that directly influence the degree of viscosity of the blood are the concentration of red blood cells (erythrocytes) and the concentration of protein molecules. By "directly influence" we mean that these factors influence blood velocity "in the same direction." If the red blood cell concentration goes up (increases), the viscosity goes up (increases). If the concentration goes down (decreases), so does the viscosity.

CHAPTER REVIEW

- The energy present at any given point in the arterial system is a combination of kinetic energy and potential energy.
- Kinetic energy is energy of motion; potential energy is energy at rest.
- Kinetic energy is determined by mass and velocity.
- Potential energy is a combination of intravascular pressure and gravitational potential energy.
- Intravascular pressure is determined by the contraction of the heart, the hydrostatic pressure, and the static filling pressure.
- Gravitational potential pressure and hydrostatic pressure are calculated by the same factors but with opposite signs.
- Energy losses can occur because of inertia, viscosity, or both.

CHAPTER

10

Arterial Pressure and Flow

In physiology, *flow* refers to the amount (volume) of fluid that moves past a given reference point within a specified unit of time. The quantity of fluid is expressed in milliliters (mL), also called cubic centimeters (cc); the unit of time is one second (s). So in talking about flow, we should be thinking in terms of milliliters or cubic centimeters per second, expressed as mL/s or cc/s respectively. The terms flow rate and volume flow express the same idea and can be used interchangeably with flow. In equations, Q is most commonly used to designate flow.

THE PRESSURE GRADIENT

We have already discussed the energy factors associated with blood flow, but why does movement (flow) occur at all? The factor most responsible for the flow of blood is the same factor responsible for the flow of any fluid: pressure, or more accurately, differences in pressure.

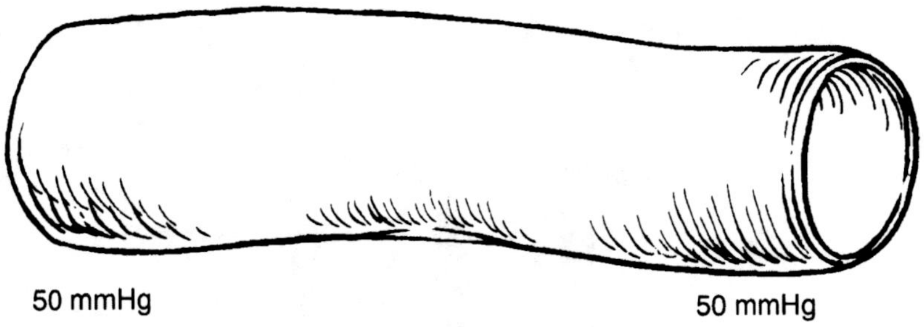

Figure 33.
There is no flow (usually) if there is no pressure gradient.

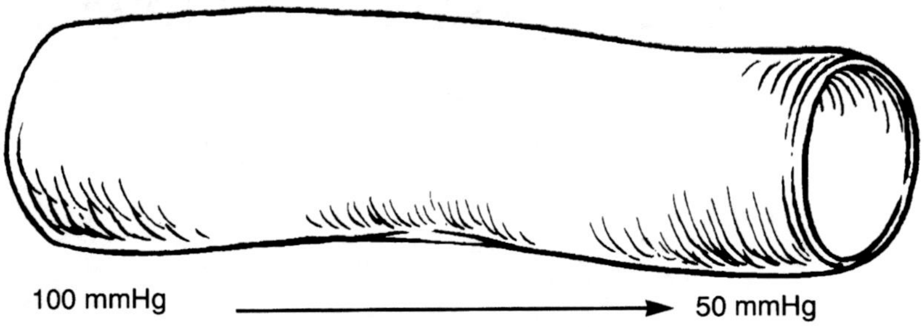

Figure 34.
Flow moves from high pressure to low pressure.

Isaac Newton's first two laws of motion explain how pressure differences are related to flow. In essence, these laws say that:

1. If no difference of pressure exists, fluid will not flow.
2. When a difference in pressure exists, fluid will flow from an area of higher pressure to an area of lower pressure.

In other words, if you have a tube filled with fluid, which, essentially, is what a blood vessel is, fluid will not move inside the tube unless there is a difference in pressure between one end and the other (Figure 33). (It is important to note here that these two statements are essentially simplifications of much more complex ideas. Therefore, as stated here, they are not always strictly true. For instance, water moving through a garden hose would contradict the first statement, because there is flow even though there is no pressure gradient within the hose itself. By the same token, the second statement, taken literally, suggests that water standing in a glass should move from the bottom of the glass [where pressure is greater] to the top [where the pressure is less] all by itself! Since we know that *that* does not occur, it becomes rather obvious that there is more to this simplified version of Newton's laws than is first apparent. Actually, the factor that keeps the water in the glass is fluid energy. Fluid *always* moves from an area of high fluid energy to one of low fluid energy, and in the glass of water the fluid energy levels are equivalent at both the top and the bottom of the glass.)

If, on the other hand, a difference exists between the pressure at one end of the tube (or vessel) and the pressure at the other end, the fluid (or blood) will move from the end with the higher pressure toward the end where pressure is lower (Figure 34).

The difference in pressure between one end of the tube and the other is called the *pressure gradient*. A pressure gradient is determined by the formula

$$\Delta P = P_1 - P_2$$

That is, the pressure at one end (P_2) is subtracted from the pressure at the other end (P_1), and the difference is the pressure gradient, which is expressed by a number (if it is known) or a letter (if it is not known) preceded by the Greek *delta*. When you see the Δ in front of a number or letter, it means difference or change in the values indicated; in the case of ΔP, a change in pressure, or pressure gradient, is represented.

If no pressure gradient exists, there is no flow. If a pressure

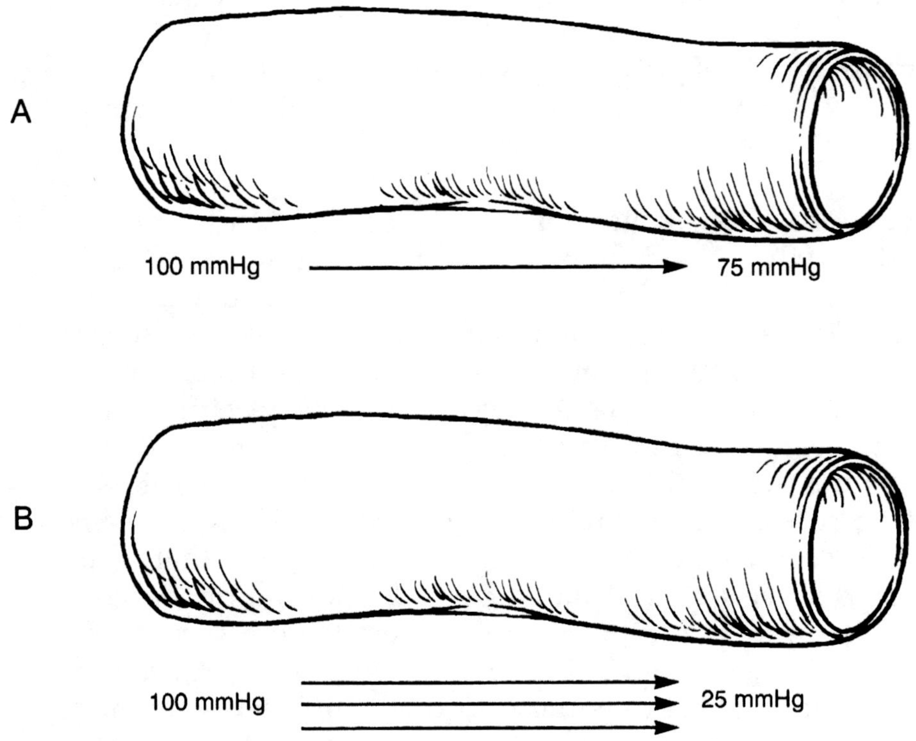

Figure 35.
The greater the pressure gradient, the greater the flow.

gradient does exist, the amount of difference affects the rate of flow. The greater the difference in pressure between two points, the faster fluid will flow between them. In other words, the greater ΔP is, the greater (faster) the flow rate.

Look at two identical tubes (Figure 35), each filled with the same type and amount of fluid but with different pressure gradients. The direction of flow in tubes A and B will be the same, but the rate of flow will differ. The pressure gradient in A is less than the gradient in B, so the flow in A will be slower.

POISEUILLE'S LAW

We have now looked at such concepts as pressure and viscosity, but we need to put them all together to see how they influence blood flow and how they are related to noninvasive testing. The laws governing the interrelationship of pressure, viscosity, and flow were first formulated by Poiseuille, a nineteenth-century physicist and physiologist. His formulas are intended to describe steady flow states, but they can be adapted to the pulsatile flow of the arterial system. Poiseuille's law can be manipulated to calculate both the effect of flow on pressure and the effect of pressure gradients on flow.

The Effect of Flow on Pressure

The best known form of *Poiseuille's law* looks rather formidable at first glance:

$$\Delta P = \frac{8\,QLV}{\pi r^4}$$

ΔP = pressure gradient across the segment being measured
Q = flow through the segment
L = length of the segment
V = viscosity of the fluid
r = radius of the segment

Notice that everything in Poiseuille's law relates to a specified segment. That is an important concept that we will come back to. For now, we will try to understand this complex equation by simplifying it. For example, you may find the equation easier to understand if it is formulated like this:

$$\Delta P = QR$$

ΔP = pressure across the segment
Q = flow across the segment
R = resistance across the segment

Although it may not seem so, this is the same concept, but it is now expressed as a multiplication problem rather than a division problem. It seems as though a lot of factors have been eliminated and a new one, R, has been added. In actuality, nothing has been added or subtracted. Look at another equation, the one for resistance, and you will see what really happened.

$$R = \frac{8LV}{\pi r^4}$$

Do you see the similarity to our original version of Poiseuille's law? All we have done is to combine all the factors that influence resistance and state them as a single entity, R.

Resistance

Before going back to Poiseuille's law, we should spend some time considering resistance. Generally speaking, resistance and flow are opposites: a high resistance means a low flow, and vice versa. All other things being equal, of two arteries of equal inside diameter, the artery with the higher resistance will have the lower flow, and the artery with the lower resistance will have the higher flow. However, all things are not necessarily equal; in the human body they often are not. The pressure gradient also affects flow. If the pressure gradient across the arterial segment with high resistance is proportionately greater than the gradient of the artery with low resistance, the arterial segment with the higher resistance will actually have the greater flow of the two.

In looking at the factors that govern resistance, we see that some influence flow directly and some indirectly. How do you tell which is which? When looking at an equation, there is a trick to remembering the relationship between the value on the left of the equal sign and the values on the right. (An equation is not in anatomic position; it is your left and your right we are referring to.)

Anything that is on the top of the right side of the equation will have a direct influence on the value that is on the left side of the equal sign. That means that any increase in the value on the

top right increases the value on the left. Similarly, any decrease in the value on the top right decreases the value on the left.

Conversely, the values that are on the bottom of the right side will have an inverse, or opposite, effect on the left side of the equation. If you increase a value on the bottom right, you will decrease the value on the left. And if you decrease a value on the bottom right, you will increase the value on the left. Therefore, these values are said to be *inversely proportional.* (This is sometimes called the indirect effect.)

Now, in looking at the factors in the resistance formula, we can determine that 8 times the flow (*F*) through a segment, the length (*L*) of the segment, and the viscosity (*V*) of the fluid within the segment will all have a direct influence on the resistance (*R*) of the segment. But π and the radius (*r*) will each have an indirect (inversely proportional) influence on this resistance.

The next step is to solve the equation. We will not assign numbers and attempt to come up with an actual value for *R*. At this point it is far more important to understand the relationships among these factors and how they influence circulation.

In solving this equation, the first thing we want to do is to eliminate those factors that never change. In a formula, any factor that never changes from one application to the next is called a *constant.* You can remove the constants from an equation without affecting the solution, so that is the first step to take.

This equation has *R* on the left side, meaning that we are going to try to "solve for *R*," that is, determine the resistance of the segment. The number 8 is always the number 8, so that is a constant and can be ignored for now. By the same token, π is a constant; it is always 3.1416 (etc.), so we can eliminate it from consideration at this point. That still leaves us with *L*, *V*, and *r*. These can represent any value and are consequently called *variables.*

We know that length has a direct influence on resistance — the longer the vessel, the more resistance it has. The length of an artery does not change under normal circumstances, so length has little influence on resistance within individual arteries. It does, however, account for differences in resistance between vessels.

For instance, collateral arteries have a higher resistance than normal arteries. In growing out, around, and back again to bypass an obstruction in a vessel, a collateral grows much longer than the original channel. This greater length is only one of several reasons why collaterals have higher resistance than normal arteries; other

reasons are discussed later in this chapter.

Viscosity of the blood can change for a number of reasons, but for all practical purposes it does not vary under normal circumstances.

That leaves us with one variable factor: the radius of the vessel. Of all the variables we have discussed, radius has the greatest effect on resistance. Look at the equation closely, and you will see that the influence of radius (*r*) on resistance is not linear, but exponential: to the fourth power of *r*. In other words, a relatively small change in radius can result in large changes in resistance. Now think of what atherosclerotic plaque deposits do: They narrow the artery; they reduce its radius.

To illustrate what happens, put some arbitrary numbers into the situation. Start with an artery that has a normal radius of 2 mm. Put a small atherosclerotic plaque in it so that the lumen is reduced to 1.75 mm. If we were to use our equation to determine the effect on resistance, the original radius would be calculated to the fourth power:

$$2 \times 2 \times 2 \times 2 = 16$$

Now, calculate the radius of 1.75 to its fourth power:

$$1.75 \times 1.75 \times 1.75 \times 1.75 = 9.38$$

What does this mean in practical terms? First, the actual reduction in size of the arterial lumen caused by this little deposit of plaque is from 2 mm to 1.75 mm, a decrease of 12.5 percent. But when we look at the <u>effect</u> of that decrease by calculating the radius to the fourth power, the numbers are dramatically different. The change from 16 to 9.38 is a 41.4 percent decrease.

Another way to look at this effect of radius on resistance is by looking at the *reciprocals* of the values we have obtained. The reciprocal of 16 is 1/16, while that of 9.38 is 1/9.38. By comparing these reciprocals, we see that 1/9.38 is 1.71 times greater than 1/16. This means that a vessel with a radius of 1.75 mm would actually have 71 percent more resistance than a vessel with a 2 mm radius.

Now you see why a change in radius that is small in actual measurement can have a major effect on vascular resistance. One reason for the high resistance present in collateral vessels is that even a well-developed collateral has a smaller lumen than the original vessel.

Returning to the simplified version of Poiseuille's law:

$$\Delta P = QR$$

Can our left/right "trick" be used to help us understand the relationships? Yes, with one small adjustment. We can always put a 1 under a value without changing the value. If we do that:
By looking at it this way, you can easily see that both flow (Q)

$$\Delta P = \frac{QR}{1}$$

through an arterial segment and resistance (R) in the segment will have a direct influence on the pressure gradient (ΔP) across the segment.

The Effect of Pressure on Flow
So far, we have discussed only the effect of flow and resistance on pressure. What about the effect of pressure gradients on flow? To determine this, we need to manipulate the Poiseuille equation again:

$$Q = \frac{\Delta P}{R}$$

This time we are looking at the flow rate (Q) as influenced by pressure gradient and resistance. By the arrangement of the equation, you can see that resistance has an inversely proportional (indirect) effect on flow. As the resistance within a segment increases, the flow decreases. Since the pressure gradient (ΔP) has a direct influence on flow, the flow through a segment will increase as the pressure gradient becomes greater. Now, if you have been following these formulas closely, you may find what looks like an inconsistency at this point.

In the version

$$\Delta P = QR$$

both the flow and the resistance directly influence the pressure gradient. Which means that increasing flow will increase the pressure gradient and increasing resistance will also increase the pressure gradient. And then we looked at the other version:

$$Q = \frac{\Delta P}{R}$$

and said that increasing the pressure gradient will increase the

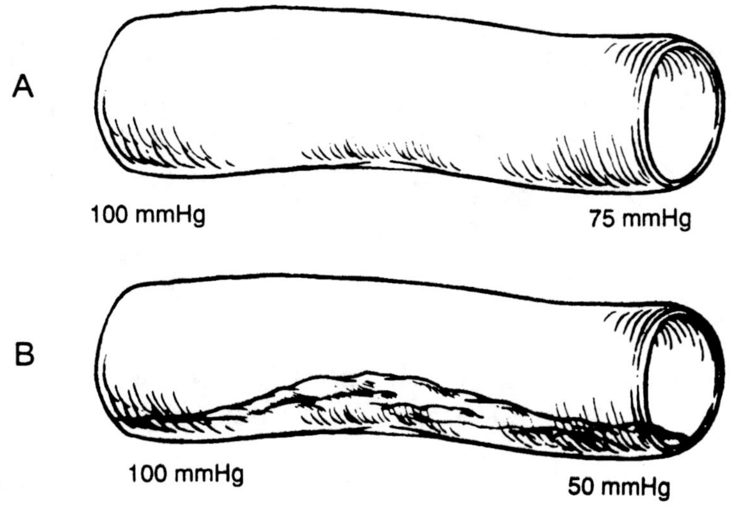

Figure 36.
Reducing the radius of the vessel increases the pressure gradient.

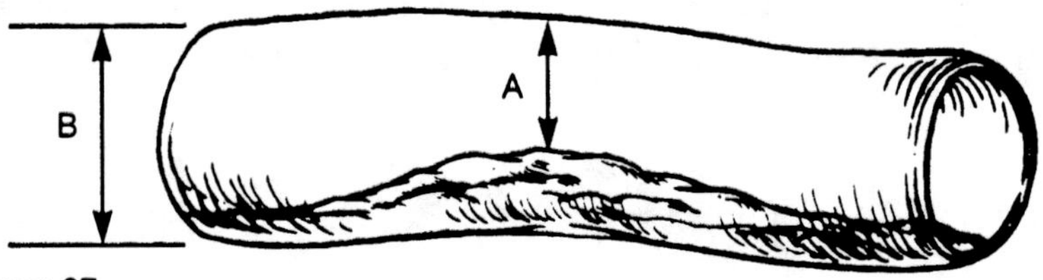

Figure 37.
To calculate the size of a stenosis in terms of percentage diameter reduction, divide A (the diameter of the remaining lumen) by B (the diameter of the original lumen) and multiply by 100. Then subtract that figure (which represents the percentage diameter that remains open to blood flow) from 100 to arrive at the percentage stenosis by diameter reduction. Here are the equations: $A/B \times 100 = X$, where X is the size of the remaining lumen expressed as a percentage of the original lumen; $100 - X = XS$, the size of the stenosis expressed as a percentage of the original lumen.

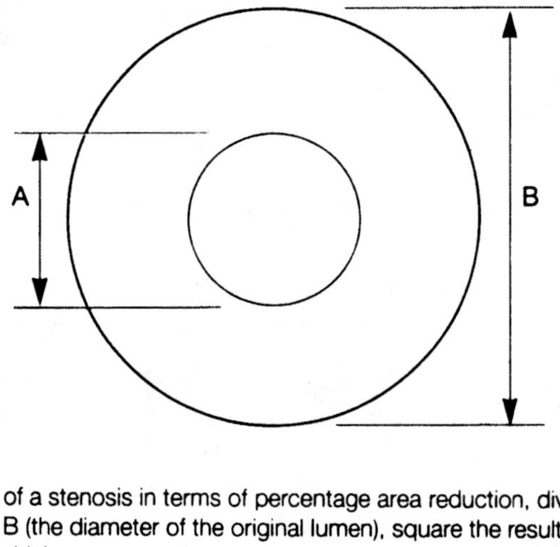

Figure 38.
To calculate the size of a stenosis in terms of percentage area reduction, divide A (the diameter of the remaining lumen) by B (the diameter of the original lumen), square the results, multiply by 100. Then subtract that figure (which represents the percentage area that remains open to blood flow) from 100 to arrive at the percentage stenosis by area reduction. Here are the equations: $(A/B)^2 \times 100 = Y$, where Y is the size of the remaining lumen expressed as a percentage of the original lumen; $100 - Y = YS$, the size of the stenosis expressed as a percentage of the original lumen.

flow. So far, so good. But this version also says that increasing the resistance will decrease the flow. It would seem that Poiseuille is contradicting himself. But there is an explanation for what is happening.

Increases in resistance do cause an increase in the pressure gradient, which does cause an increase in flow, even though increases in resistance will cause a decrease in flow. The explanation is that different factors have different degrees of influence at different times.

Suppose you place an obstruction in a blood-vessel segment, thereby decreasing its radius. This reduction in radius causes an increased resistance in the vessel which, in turn, causes an increase in the pressure gradient across the segment (Figure 36).

In the beginning, the increase in pressure gradient has the dominant effect on the flow rate. The body tries to deliver the same amount of blood across the obstruction that it was delivering when the artery was wide open. To accomplish that with the opening being smaller, the flow rate has to increase. Eventually, however, the distal circulation becomes compromised to the point where the increased resistance in the segment is enough to reduce the flow passing through the obstruction. When the obstruction becomes sufficiently severe to reduce the diameter of the vessel by 50 percent (or the area by 75 percent), it becomes a *flow-reducing* or *hemodynamically significant* lesion.

Let's take a minute to discuss the two ways of indicating the size of a stenosis: diameter reduction and area reduction. If you section an artery along its length and look into the lumen longitudinally to determine its size, you are trying to determine *diameter reduction*. This is done by comparing the lumen at its narrowest part with its normal width and multiplying the number by 100 (see Figure 37). But if you section the same artery transversely across its narrowest point, you can measure its *reduction in area*. You again compare the normal lumen with the reduced lumen and multiply by 100, but this time you also would square the comparison of the two lumens (Figure 38). These two terms—diameter reduction and area reduction—are not interchangeable. They are much the same as comparing a linear measurement across two rooms (the diameter reduction) and the square footage of two rooms (the area reduction).

CHAPTER REVIEW

- Flow (flow rate; volume flow) occurs primarily because of pressure gradients (differences in pressure). Generally, a pressure gradient must exist for flow to occur.
- When a pressure gradient is present, flow moves from the area of higher pressure to the area of lower pressure; the greater the pressure gradient, the greater the flow rate.
- Poiseuille's law explains the interrelationship among pressure, viscosity, and flow.
- Poiseuille's law is most commonly written as

$$\Delta P = \frac{8QLV}{\pi r^4}$$

It can also be expressed more simply as

$$\Delta P = QR \text{ or as } Q = \frac{\Delta P}{R}$$

- Generally, resistance and flow are opposite factors; when one increases, the other decreases, and vice versa.
- Resistance is expressed by the formula

$$R = \frac{8LV}{\pi r^4}$$

- The radius of a vessel has the greatest effect on resistance.
- An obstruction producing 50 percent diameter reduction (or 75 percent area reduction) is considered a flow-reducing, or hemodynamically significant, lesion.

Only one aspect of arterial hemodynamics remains to be covered. In discussing the carotid bulb, we touched briefly on the topic of pressoreceptors as a mechanism for controlling heart rate. Pressoreceptors are also one of several mechanisms for regulating the flow of blood in the body.

CHAPTER

11

Mechanisms of Control

The body has a number of methods for controlling and regulating blood flow. Both the velocity of the flow and the area to which it is directed can be controlled. There are two aspects to this control: First, blood must be kept moving through the body; that is, circulation must be maintained. Second, the volume of blood being moved must be controlled; that is, the circulation must be varied. The matter is not so simple as having one mechanism for maintaining the circulation and one for varying it. Both these aspects require a complex network of mechanisms working together.

We have already discussed most of the factors that maintain the circulation, including the pumping action of the heart, the energy of the blood flow, and pressure gradients within the vessels. Now let us look at the factors that determine the volume of blood flowing in the circulation. This control has two aspects: (1) regulating the volume of blood moving throughout the circulatory system, and (2) regulating the volume of blood moving into and out of any given area within the body.

CARDIAC MINUTE OUTPUT

We said in Chapter 10 that blood flow is measured in volume units per unit of time, generally milliters per second (mL/s). When we talk about varying the volume of blood moving throughout the circulatory system, we are talking about the rate of flow per minute or second, not the quantity of blood being moved. Blood must move at different flow rates to meet different needs, or demands, of the body. The two principal factors that control this variation in volume are cardiac minute output and peripheral resistance.

You can figure out the definition of *cardiac minute output* for yourself: It is the volume (output) of blood being ejected by the heart over a period of 1 minute. (This term is often shortened to just "cardiac output.") Two factors determine cardiac output: stroke volume and heart rate.

Stroke Volume

Stroke volume is the volume of blood that enters the aorta with each contraction of the left ventricle. If we express this as an equation, it looks like this:

$$CMO = SV \times HR$$

CMO = cardiac minute output
SV = stroke volume
HR = heart rate

In looking at this equation, we see that both stroke volume and heart rate have a direct influence on cardiac minute output (see Chapter 10). Increasing either of these factors will increase output, and decreasing either will lower it. That concept is easy to grasp. If you make the heart pump more times each minute, more blood will move out into the arterial system each minute. Or, if you increase the amount of blood moving through the aorta with each heartbeat, more blood will be entering the arterial system each minute. Increases in blood volume lead to increases in systemic blood pressure, and vice versa. In other words, factors that influence blood volume also exert influence on blood pressure.

The stroke volume is related to the strength of the contraction of the left ventricle. So, anything that increases or decreases the contractile strength of the left ventricle will automatically increase or decrease stroke volume. A number of factors affect ventricular

contractile strength, including chemical and neural (nerve-generated) influences. One of the most dominant influences is sheerly mechanical. Remember that the left ventricle, which is the largest and strongest of the heart's four chambers, is composed mainly of a muscle layer called the myocardium. The state of the myocardium exerts a mechanical influence on stroke volume.

Muscles are like rubber bands in that they stretch and contract. If you stretch a rubber band just a little and then let it go, the "snap" will be fairly weak. If you pull the rubber band as tautly as you can, the snap when you let it go will be strong. The same is true of muscles. If a muscle is stretched tightly before a contraction, the contraction will be strong. The less the stretch, the weaker the contraction.

In the heart, the amount by which the myocardium stretches is related to the amount of blood that fills the chambers. The more blood in the ventricle, the more it expands, the more tightly the myocardium stretches, and the stronger the contraction as the ventricle empties.

However, there is a limit to the heart muscle's ability to stretch. To go back to the rubber band example: If I keep stretching the rubber band to its limit, or if I try to stretch it beyond its limit, eventually I will wear it out. Its elasticity will be diminished, and even if I pull it out as far as it will go, the snap will be weak. The same thing is true of the heart. Once a certain degree of stretch has been reached, further stretching actually appears to diminish the effectiveness of the contraction. This principle of stretch and contractive force is called Starling's law of the heart, or simply *Starling's law.*

Heart Rate

A number of different mechanisms also control the heart rate, but one is dominant, the effect of pressoreceptors. *Receptors* are sensory nerve endings that respond to different types of stimuli, such as light, sound, or the presence of certain chemicals. *Pressoreceptors,* sometimes called baroreceptors, are sensitive to changes in pressure. In discussing the cardiopulmonary circulation, we mentioned important pressoreceptors in the carotid sinus and in the aortic arch. Stimulation of receptors in either location will decrease the heart rate.

Carotid massage or any form of accidental or intentional pressure on the carotid sinus will slow the heart. Normally,

however, pressoreceptors in the carotid sinus and the aorta respond to pressure changes in the arteries where they are located. If pressure increases in either artery, more electrochemical impulses are sent to the vagus nerve, causing the heart rate to slow; at the same time, fewer impulses are sent to the nerves that increase the heart rate. The net effect is a reflexive slowing of the heart rate. (The next time your favorite TV sleuth says that the strangling victim died of "vagal inhibition," you will know what that means.)

Conversely, if blood pressure in the aorta or the carotid artery were suddenly to decrease, a series of events would be set in motion to increase the heart rate. There would be less stimulation of the pressoreceptors, the nerves that increase the heart rate would receive more impulses, and those that slow the heart would receive fewer. The net result would be to raise the heart rate. (Both of these explanations greatly simplify the complex neural and hormonal activities that actually occur.)

Another group of receptors also affect the heart rate. These *exteroreceptors* are sensitive to the immediate external environment. For instance, nerve receptors in the skin respond to environmental temperature changes in such a way that the heart rate will drop at freezing temperatures and increase when it is hot.

Chemicals that are released into the blood during different emotional states also act to regulate the heart rate. When you are angry or frightened, your heart beats faster than when you are relaxed or enjoying yourself. Hormones called *neurotransmitters* are involved in these responses. The most familiar of these is *epinephrine* (adrenaline). You may have said "My adrenaline was up" to describe a situation in which you were very angry, under extreme stress, or otherwise "ready for action." Epinephrine directly affects the heart rate; the more epinephrine present, the faster the heart will beat.

Finally, exercise influences the heart rate. The more active the body is, the greater the demand of the tissues for oxygenated blood. A multitude of complex signals "tell" the heart that you have increased your activity level, and it responds by beating faster. If you are out playing tennis, your body requires a heart rate considerably faster than it needs if you are lying in bed reading a book—even a very exciting book.

Now that you have had a very simplified overview of cardiac minute output and the factors that control it, we can discuss the other major control mechanism, peripheral resistance.

PERIPHERAL RESISTANCE

Peripheral resistance is controlled by the expansion (*vasodilatation*) and contraction (*vasoconstriction*) of the small vessels of the periphery, the arterioles and the arterial capillaries. The arterioles can expand or contract over a fairly wide range to regulate the volume of blood that goes to any body area or organ.

A number of different factors affect vasoconstriction and vasodilatation. The brain, acting through the autonomous nervous system, exerts continual fine control. Some nerves dilate the vessels, some may either dilate or constrict them, depending on which neurotransmitters are released. Pressoreceptors in the carotid sinus and the aortic arch exert influence all the way to the capillaries, as do other pressoreceptors elsewhere in the body.

The nerves that influence muscles in the vessel walls to expand or contract them respond to many local stimuli. Changes in the blood's content of different chemicals have a major effect on arterial size. In response to hypoxia, a reduction in the oxygen level of the blood, the arterioles will dilate. They will also dilate in response to hypercapnia, which is an increase in the blood's level of carbon dioxide.

Another local factor that stimulates changes in the diameter of the arterioles is localized ischemia, a reduction in the local supply of oxygenated blood. If the arterial blood supply to a body area is restricted or interrupted, the tissue becomes ischemic. Substances called ischemic metabolites accumulate in the ischemic tissue. Their presence causes discomfort, but their main function is to alert special receptors and thereby induce vasodilatation.

Once the obstruction to blood flow has been removed, blood literally floods the area through the maximally dilated vessels. This increase of flow to a body part is called *reactive hyperemia.* Hyper- means increased, and *emia* (from the word heme, for blood) means being supplied with blood. You have probably experienced reactive hyperemia if you have ever had your blood pressure taken. When the cuff is inflated above systolic pressure, no blood enters your arm, and the buildup of ischemic metabolites makes it hurt. This discomfort disappears rapidly after the cuff is deflated and reactive hyperemia brings blood to the arm to wash away the accumulated metabolites.

Can you see how peripheral resistance regulates blood flow? Recall that without pressure gradients blood would not move through the vessels, and that the greater the pressure gradient, the

greater the blood flow. By expanding and contracting specific blood vessels, the body regulates the proportion of the total circulating blood that goes to any portion of the body at a given time.

Some parts of the body, such as the brain, have a relatively constant flow rate. Other areas have much more variable needs. For instance, if you are sitting in an easy chair, your leg muscles need less blood flow than they do if you are walking around the room. Your leg muscles will need even more blood if you are climbing stairs, and still more if you are running. Similarly, your digestive organs need more blood just after a heavy meal than they do a few hours later. (Can you relate this information to the caution not to swim right after a meal?) These variations in blood flow are almost entirely a function of peripheral resistance.

Another factor that contributes to peripheral resistance is the viscosity of the blood. But, again, blood viscosity does not vary much under normal circumstances. Consequently, the regulation of the blood flow to meet minute-by-minute needs of different body areas is governed mainly by the diameter of the arterioles.

CHAPTER REVIEW

- The two principal control mechanisms governing blood volume changes within the body are the cardiac minute output and the peripheral resistance.
- Cardiac minute output is the volume of blood ejected by the heart in 1 minute.
- Cardiac output is determined by the stroke volume (amount of blood ejected with each beat) and the heart rate (number of beats per minute).
- Receptors are sensory nerve endings that respond to a variety of stimuli. Pressoreceptors (also called baroreceptors) respond to changes in pressure; exteroreceptors are sensitive to their immediate environment.
- Stimulation of pressoreceptors in the carotid bulb and aortic arch causes reflex bradycardia.
- Peripheral resistance is controlled by the constriction (vasoconstriction) and expansion (vasodilatation) of the arterioles and arterial capillaries.

SECTION FIVE

Venous Hemodynamics

How blood moves through the arterial network is only half the picture, although "half" is somewhat misleading. At any given time, about 75 percent of the circulating blood in your body is moving through the venous system instead of the arterial. So, understanding the mechanisms by which venous return to the heart is accomplished is crucial to understanding the physiology of the vascular system.

You have learned how oxygenated blood is distributed to the tissues and how the volume of this blood sent to any given area is regulated. But in order for the blood to move from the heart to the periphery, it must first be returned to the heart. That means that something must be pushing it through the venous portion of the circulatory system. That something is not a single entity but a group of somethings working together. Like arterial hemodynamics, venous hemodynamics depend on the interaction of a number of factors.

CHAPTER

12

Venous Pressure and Flow

The first characteristic we associated with arterial flow was pulsatility. At that time we said that the direct influence of the pulsing heart on the venous system is minimal. Most veins do not pulsate, but there are two full and one partial exception to that rule. Because of their relationship to the heart, the internal jugular vein and the subclavian vein are normally pulsatile. The axillary vein is sometimes pulsatile and sometimes not, depending on the individual. Pulsatility in the axillary vein is not considered abnormal, but, rather, an individual variation.

If nonpulsatility is normal in all but the great veins, is some characteristic of flow typical of veins? Yes. The characteristic of flow typical of veins is phasicity.

PHASICITY

The term *phasicity*, in reference to the venous system, refers to the ebb and flow that occurs in normal veins in response to

respiration. All deep veins normally exhibit phasicity, even those that are somewhat pulsatile. If you were listening to (auscultating) the internal jugular vein, for instance, you would expect to hear a sound that was both pulsatile and phasic. Respiration has this ebb/flow influence because unlike the strong-walled arteries, veins are collapsible (see Chapter 3).

The two phases of respiration are *inspiration* (breathing in) and *expiration* (breathing out). The way in which the blood moves in phase with respiration differs according to the part of the body affected and the position in which the body is placed. As an example, we can look at venous return from the lower limbs in an upright body.

Venous Return from the Lower Extremities

When a body is standing upright, breathing produces pressure gradients that influence the movement of venous blood. As the lungs fill with air during inspiration, the thoracic cavity expands. When the thorax expands, the diaphragm drops; consequently the abdominal cavity becomes smaller. The veins located within the chest and abdomen are affected by these changes in pressure.

As the thoracic cavity gets larger, pressure within it decreases, and pressure within the right atrium and the thoracic portion of the vena cava is also reduced. At the same time, the abdominal cavity is getting smaller, raising the pressure within the abdomen and the abdominal veins. You have already learned that fluids move from areas of high pressure to areas of low pressure, so you can deduce that during inspiration, more venous blood from the lower body will move into the thoracic area, which has the lower pressure.

With expiration, the process reverses itself. When the lungs expel air, the thoracic cavity becomes smaller and the abdominal cavity grows larger. Now the intraabdominal pressure is lower than the intrathoracic pressure, and less blood will move from the veins of the lower extremities into the veins of the chest.

However, as we said at the outset, the position of the body influences the effects of respiration on venous flow. Consider what happens to venous flow in your lower extremities when you are supine (lying on your back).

Even when you are supine, you expand your chest when you inhale. But now the space in which your chest can expand is limited by the surface on which you are lying. When you fill your

lungs with air, they push your posterior thorax against this surface, compressing the vena cava so that blood cannot enter it. Venous flow from the lower extremities will diminish. When you exhale, you release the compression on the vena cava, allowing blood from the lower extremities to enter it once more. So, when you are lying down, respiration has an effect opposite to what occurs when you are standing up.

Venous Return from the Upper Extremities

Respiration also affects venous return from the upper extremities, but to a lesser extent than it affects the lower body. Again, phasicity in the upper-extremity veins also can vary according to circumstances. If you are listening to a brachial vein, for instance, inspiration may produce either a reduced sound or an increased sound. If the lowered, or negative, intrathoracic pressure causes more blood to move from the brachial vein to the subclavian, sound from the brachial vein will increase. Sometimes, however, expansion of the lungs on inspiration will physically compress the subclavian vein. When this happens, less venous blood will move from the chest into the arms, and sound in the brachial vein will diminish.

The importance of all this is that you should be able to detect phasic changes in all the deep veins in relationship to breathing.

HYDROSTATIC PRESSURE

In Chapter 10 you learned a little about hydrostatic pressure in relation to arterial physiology. The principles discussed there also apply to venous hemodynamics. As you have just learned, changes in pressure in various parts of the body partially determine the movement of arterial blood. Changes in pressure within different veins also influence the movement of venous blood. So does the relationship between different types of pressure and energy, specifically hydrostatic pressure.

As stated earlier, *hydrostatic pressure* is the pressure exerted by fluid within a closed system. The equation we used for determining hydrostatic pressure is:

$$HP = \rho g h$$

HP = hydrostatic pressure
ρ = specific gravity of the blood
g = acceleration due to gravity
h = height above a specified reference point

To review briefly: We said that the hydrostatic pressure in the vessel, together with the muscular contraction of the heart and the static filling pressure of the blood, determined the intravascular pressure. The static filling pressure has a negligible effect. The muscular contraction of the heart (which can also be called dynamic pressure) chiefly affects the arterial system, not the venous. That leaves hydrostatic pressure as the primary factor in determining intravascular pressure within the venous circulation.

Hydrostatic pressure varies with position. For instance, when you are lying down, there is virtually no hydrostatic pressure in your legs, since they are at the same level as the right atrium, which has a pressure of around zero. But when you stand up, the situation changes drastically. When you are upright, the veins of the lower extremity represent a long tube or column of fluid. The hydrostatic pressure in that tube is considerable.

As an example: Say that in a 6-foot person who is supine the venous pressure at the level of the ankle is about 10 mmHg. When that person stands up, the ankle venous pressure rises to 112 mmHg. As this occcurs, the veins of the legs dilate to accept the blood that is pooling in them. In fact, it is estimated that about 250 mL of blood shifts to the legs when a person who is lying down stands up.

In Chapter 13, we will discuss the mechanisms that interact to move this venous blood out of the legs, back to the heart, then out again into the arterial system.

CHAPTER REVIEW

- Phasicity—the ebb and flow of blood that occurs in response to respiration—is a flow characteristic common to all deep veins.
- Pulsatility is abnormal in veins, with the exception of the internal jugular and subclavian veins and, in some individuals, the axillary vein. (To be normal, these veins should also exhibit phasicity.)
- When the body is supine, inspiration decreases the flow of venous blood out of the lower extremities; expiration increases venous return to the heart.
- When the body is in the standing position, inspiration increases venous return to the heart; expiration decreases it.
- Hydrostatic pressure—the pressure exerted by fluid within a closed system—varies with position.

CHAPTER

13

The Venous Valves and the Leg Muscles

If you think over what you learned in the previous chapter, you will recognize a potentially troublesome factor in venous return from the lower extremities to the heart: gravity. In a standing person, the effect of gravity is substantial. Although moving venous blood from the head to the heart is no problem—gravity, in fact, actually helps—moving blood from the ankle to the heart, against gravity, is a real challenge. Two factors work together to overcome this challenge: the venous valves we described in Chapter 4, and the muscles of the legs.

FUNCTION OF THE VENOUS VALVES

The venous valves play an indirect role in moving blood, rather like a police officer directing traffic at an intersection. The officer can point at a waiting car, indicating that it should move, and he can indicate the direction, but this in itself does not cause the car to move.

Basically, venous valves direct flow. They keep the blood moving back toward the heart in both the deep and the superficial veins. In the perforating veins, the valves direct the flow from the superficial to the deep veins. If the venous valves are functioning normally, they prevent *reflux*, or backflow, of venous blood by trapping blood in their cusps, or leaflets, as they close. Venous valves open and close in conjunction with the action of the muscles.

Going back to our traffic example, the police officer points at a car and indicates that it should go through the intersection. For the car to do so, however, the driver must apply power to propel the car. In the veins, this propulsion is provided by muscle contraction.

THE MUSCLE PUMP

In defining deep veins versus superficial veins we said that deep veins are situated not just under the skin but deeply under the fascia. In the extremities, the deep veins are surrounded by muscles. As these muscles contract, they squeeze the veins within them. Muscles do not remain permanently contracted; to function they must alternately contract and relax. This alternating contraction/relaxation "milks" the venous blood, propelling it up the leg. As the muscle pump moves the blood, the valves direct its flow back to the heart.

In the introduction to this section, we said that about 75 percent of the circulating blood is within the venous system at any given time. A large percentage of that venous blood is in the lower half of the body. If the muscle pump is not activated while the legs are in a dependent position, that is, while you are sitting or standing, blood will pool in the lower extremities. If an insufficient volume of venous blood is being returned to the heart, an insufficient amount will be sent to the lungs to be oxygenated. One result of this is that insufficient oxygen will be sent to the brain. This leads to syncope: In other words, you faint.

That is an extreme example. Usually, venous pooling is not severe enough to lead to significant hypoxia. However, it does lead to edema (swelling) at the ankles. If you take a long plane trip and stay seated throughout, your feet and ankles will become quite swollen. If you get up and walk around, the edema will not be as severe. If, in addition, you flex your legs frequently to activate the muscle pump, you may have little edema or none at all.

Walking, obviously, activates the muscles in the lower extremities. However, these muscles can be activated while sitting or standing still. Alternately tightening and relaxing the calf and thigh muscles will help propel the venous blood along its path, even while your body is inactive.

By the way, the muscle pump of the leg has a variety of names. Different texts and journal articles refer to it as the muscle pump, calf pump, calf muscle pump, soleal pump, leg muscle pump, venous pump, and many other names. The most fanciful name is the venous heart. Though it sounds romantic, this name has some validity: After all, the real heart is a large muscle that pumps blood, just like the muscles surrounding the deep veins.

Back at the intersection, the interaction of the traffic cop and the car's motor kept traffic moving, and moving in the right direction. In the venous system, it is the interaction of the venous valves and the muscle pump that keeps venous blood moving, and moving in the right direction. When these two elements are working properly, the veins in the lower extremities can empty so effectively that emptying is actually complete.

For instance, say that while a person is standing still, he or she has an ankle venous pressure of 90 mmHg. Now that person begins to exercise the leg muscles, thereby activating the muscle pump system. If the valves and the pump are functioning properly, the ankle venous pressure will fall to 30 mmHg or even lower—possibly even to 0 mmHg.

Even though the action of the muscle pump works mainly on the deep veins, it has some influence on the superficial veins as well. Strong muscle contractions in the leg put a slight degree of compression on the surrounding superficial veins also, propelling the blood in those veins upward.

CHAPTER REVIEW

- The two factors that interact to move venous blood out of the lower extremities and back to the heart are the venous valves and the leg muscles.
- Venous valves are designed to direct, rather than propel, venous blood.
- Deep and superficial valves direct blood toward the heart; perforating/communicating vein valves direct blood from the superficial veins toward the deep veins.
- The calf muscle pump acts by alternately contracting and relaxing around the veins.
- An effective valve/muscle pump interaction can move large quantities of blood out of the lower extremities and is even capable of completely emptying the lower extremity veins.

Suggested Readings

Clemente CD: *Anatomy: A Regional Atlas of the Human Body*, 6th edition. Lippincott Williams and Wilkins, 2011.

Gray H: *Gray's Anatomy*, 41st edition. Churchill Livingstone, 2015.

Kupinski AM: *Diagnostic Medical Sonography*. Lippincott Williams and Wilkins, 2012.

Owen CA, Strandness DE: *ScoreCards for Vascular Technology: A Q&A Flashcard Study System for Vascular Technology*, 2nd edition. Davies, 2016.

Pellerito JS, Polak JF: *Introduction to Vascular Ultrasonography*, 7th edition. Elsevier/Saunders, 2019.

Ridgway D, Bean B, Owen CA, Strandness DE: *Vascular Technology Review*, 4th edition. Davies, 2014.

Rumwell C, McPharlin M: *Vascular Technology: An Illustrated Review*, 5th edition. Davies, 2014.

Size GP, Lozanski L, Russo T: *Inside Ultrasound Vascular Reference Guide: The Complete Guide to Vascular Disease, Non-Invasive Testing and Interpretation*. Inside Ultrasound, 2013.

Talbot SR, Oliver MA, Strandness DE: *Venous Imaging Techniques*, 2nd edition. Davies, 2007.

Index

Application for CME Credit

Vascular Anatomy and Physiology

An Introductory Text

This continuing medical educational (CME) activity is approved for 5 hours of credit by the Society of Diagnostic Medical Sonography. This credit may be applied as follows:

- Sonographers and technologists may apply these hours toward the CME requirements of the ARDMS, ARRT, and/or CCI, as well as to the CME requirements of IAC and AIUM for technologists and sonographers in facilities accredited by those organizations.

- Physicians may apply a certain maximum number of SDMS-approved credit hours toward the CME requirements of the IAC and AIUM for accreditation of diagnostic facilities. (Be sure to confirm current requirements with the pertinent organizations.) Physicians who are registered sonographers or technologists may apply all of these hours toward the CME requirements of the ARDMS, ARRT, and/or CCI. SDMS-approved credit is not applicable toward the AMA Physician's Recognition Award.

If you have any questions whatsoever about CME requirements that affect you, please contact the responsible organization directly for current information. CME requirements can and sometimes do change.

OBJECTIVES OF THE ACTIVITY

Upon completion of this educational activity, you will be able to:

1 Identify the gross anatomy of the central and peripheral arterial and venous systems.

2 Describe the physiology and fluid dynamics of the central and peripheral circulation.

3 Use anatomic terminology to describe planes, areas, regions, direction, and location.

HOW TO OBTAIN CME CREDIT

To apply for credit, please do all of the following:

1 Read and study the book and complete the interactive exercises it contains.

2 Photocopy and complete the following application form, evaluation questionnaire (you grade us!), and answer sheet.

3 Make copies of the completed application, evaluation, and answer sheet for your records and then return the originals together with payment of the administrative processing fee to the following address:

Davies Publishing, Inc.
CME Coordinator
32 South Raymond Avenue, Suite 4
Pasadena, California 91105-1961

Or you can fax your application, answer sheet, evaluation form, and credit card number, expiration date, and 3- or 4-digit security code to 1-626-792-5308, or email to cme@DaviesPublishing.com.

We grade quizzes within 24 hours of receipt and will email your certificate. Questions? Please call us at 626-792-3046.

4 If more than one person will be applying for credit, be sure to photocopy the applicant information, evaluation form, and CME quiz so that you always have the original on hand for use.

APPLICANT INFORMATION

Name ____________________ Birthdate ____________

Current credentials ____________________

Home Address ____________________

City/State/Zip ____________________

Telephone ____________ Email address ____________

ARDMS # ________ ARRT # ________ CCI# ________ SDMS # ________

☐ I purchased the book myself (new, not used). ☐ I borrowed the book or purchased it used.

Check Enclosed ☐

Credit Card # ____________ Exp. Date ________ 3 or 4 digit code ________

Signature certifying your completion of the activity and authorizing payment:

____

NOTE: The original purchaser of this CME activity is entitled to submit this CME application for an administrative fee of $39.50. Please enclose a check payable to Davies Publishing, Inc., or include credit card information with your application. Others may also submit applications for CME credits by completing the activity for an administrative fee of $49.50. The CME administrative fee helps to defray the cost of processing, evaluating, and maintaining a record of your application and the credit you earn. Fees may change without notice. For the current fee, call us at 626-792-3046, email us at **cme@DaviesPublishing.com**, or write to us at the aforementioned address. We will be happy to help!

Evaluation—You Grade Us!

Please let us know what you think of *Vascular Anatomy and Physiology*. Participating in this quality survey is a requirement for CME applicants, and it benefits future readers by ensuring that current readers are satisfied and, if not, that their comments and opinions are heard and taken into account. Your opinion counts!

1 Why did you purchase *Vascular Anatomy and Physiology*? (Circle primary reason.)

Registry review Course text Clinical reference CME activity

2 Have you used *Vascular Anatomy and Physiology* for other reasons, too? (Circle all that apply.)

Registry review Course text Clinical reference CME activity

3 To what extent did *Vascular Anatomy and Physiology* meet its stated objectives and your needs? (Circle one.)

Greatly Moderately Minimally Insignificantly

4 The content of *Vascular Anatomy and Physiology* was (circle one):

Just right Too basic Too advanced

5 The quality of the questions and explanations was mainly (circle one):

Excellent Good Fair Poor

6 The manner in which *Vascular Anatomy and Physiology* presents the material is mainly (circle one):

Excellent Good Fair Poor

7 If you used this book to prepare for the registry exam, did you also use other materials or take any exam-preparation courses?

No Yes (please specify what materials and courses)

____

____

8 If you used this book for a course, please name the course, the instructor's name, the name of the school or program, and any other textbooks you may have used.

Course/Instructor/School or program: ____________________

____

Other textbooks: ______________________________

____

9 What did you like best about *Vascular Anatomy and Physiology*?

____

____

10 What did you like least about *Vascular Anatomy and Physiology*?

____

____

11 If you used *Vascular Anatomy and Physiology* to prepare for your registry exam in vascular technology, did you pass?

Yes No Haven't yet taken it

12 May we quote any of your comments in our catalogs or promotional material?

Yes No

Further comment . . .

____

____

____

____

ANSWER SHEET

Circle the correct answers below and return this sheet together with the application information and evaluation form to Davies Publishing, Inc., or fax to 1-626-792-5308. Passing criterion is 70% for attempt 1 and (for those who do not pass on the first attempt) 75% for attempts 2 and 3. The applicant may not have more than 3 attempts to pass.

1.	A B C D E	21.	A B C D E	41.	A B C D E
2.	A B C D E	22.	A B C D E	42.	A B C D E
3.	A B C D E	23.	A B C D E	43.	A B C D E
4.	A B C D E	24.	A B C D E	44.	A B C D E
5.	A B C D E	25.	A B C D E	45.	A B C D E
6.	A B C D E	26.	A B C D E	46.	A B C D E
7.	A B C D E	27.	A B C D E	47.	A B C D E
8.	A B C D E	28.	A B C D E	48.	A B C D E
9.	A B C D E	29.	A B C D E	49.	A B C D E
10.	A B C D E	30.	A B C D E	50.	A B C D E
11.	A B C D E	31.	A B C D E		
12.	A B C D E	32.	A B C D E		
13.	A B C D E	33.	A B C D E		
14.	A B C D E	34.	A B C D E		
15.	A B C D E	35.	A B C D E		
16.	A B C D E	36.	A B C D E		
17.	A B C D E	37.	A B C D E		
18.	A B C D E	38.	A B C D E		
19.	A B C D E	39.	A B C D E		
20.	A B C D E	40.	A B C D E		

CME QUIZ

Please answer the following questions after you have completed the CME activity. There is one best answer for each question. Circle it on the answer sheet. Passing criterion is 70% for attempt 1 and (for those who do not pass on the first attempt) 75% for attempts 2 and 3. The applicant may not have more than 3 attempts to pass.

1. Which of the following arteries is NOT found in the lower extremity?
   a. profunda femoris
   b. peroneal
   c. anterior tibial
   d. internal pudendal
   e. superficial femoral

2. Which of the following statements about venous valves is true?
   a. Venous valves assist flow back to the heart.
   b. Venous valves are found in the deep rather than superficial venous system.
   c. Venous valves are found only in the legs, not the arms.
   d. Venous valves are more prevalent in the superficial veins.
   e. Venous valves enhance the effect of gravity on flow in the deep veins of the legs.

3. Which adjective refers to the walls of a cavity?
   a. visceral
   b. epithelial
   c. parietal
   d. intimal
   e. cavital

4. Approximately what percentage of circulating blood volume is within the venous portion of the circulation at any one time?
   a. 50%
   b. 75%
   c. 25%
   d. 100%
   e. 15%

5. Which two factors determine the cardiac minute output?
   a. stroke volume and heart size
   b. heart size and blood viscosity
   c. heart rate and stroke volume
   d. heart size and heart rate
   e. stroke volume and blood viscosity

6. Where is the common femoral vein located?
   a. inferior to the inguinal ligament
   b. posterior to the medial malleolus
   c. anterior to the lateral malleolus
   d. superior to the inguinal ligament
   e. lateral to the adductor canal

7. The first branch of the right subclavian artery is the:

   a. basilar artery
   b. right axillary artery
   c. right vertebral artery
   d. right common carotid artery
   e. innominate artery

8. Which of the following is a true statement?

   a. The ears are located on the ventral aspect of the head.
   b. The great toe is lateral to the third digit of the foot.
   c. The nose is on the dorsal surface of the head.
   d. Digit #3 of the hand is medial to digit #5.
   e. The second digit of the foot is medial to the fifth digit.

9. What is the name of the heart valve through which blood passes from the right atrium to the right ventricle?

   a. mitral valve
   b. bicuspid valve
   c. aortic valve
   d. tricuspid valve
   e. pulmonary valve

10. What is the name of the superficial vein on the lateral aspect of the arm?

    a. basilic vein
    b. small saphenous vein
    c. cephalic vein
    d. lateral perforating vein
    e. great saphenous vein

11. Which plane divides the body into front and back halves?

    a. sagittal plane
    b. horizontal plane
    c. coronal plane
    d. transverse plane
    e. median sagittal plane

12. Which of the following pulses is normally palpated on or near the foot?

    a. common femoral artery pulse
    b. popliteal artery pulse
    c. common iliac artery pulse
    d. pudendal artery pulse
    e. peroneal artery pulse

13. Another name for the chest cavity is:

    a. parietal cavity
    b. thoracic cavity
    c. truncal cavity
    d. cardiac cavity
    e. visceral cavity

14. The three terminal branches of the ophthalmic artery are the:

   a. frontal, supraorbital, and infraorbital arteries
   b. nasal, frontal, infraorbital arteries
   c. supraorbital, frontal, and facial arteries
   d. facial, nasal, and supraorbital arteries
   e. nasal, frontal, and supraorbital arteries

15. Which of the following is a deep vein?

   a. femoral vein
   b. great saphenous vein
   c. basilic vein
   d. small saphenous vein
   e. cephalic vein

16. A red blood cell leaves the left ventricle and continues down the thoracic and abdominal aorta to the right lower extremity. Through which of the following arteries would it NOT pass on its way to the foot?

   a. common iliac
   b. popliteal
   c. common femoral
   d. internal iliac
   e. external iliac

17. The following term is used to describe the tendency of things to maintain their status quo:

   a. kinetic energy
   b. inertia
   c. viscosity
   d. potential energy
   e. resistance

18. According to Poiseuille's law, what effect would there be on the pressure gradient across a segment if you decreased the radius of the segment?

   a. There would be no effect.
   b. The pressure gradient would increase.
   c. The pressure gradient would decrease.
   d. The pressure gradient would either decrease or increase, depending on the individual artery.
   e. It is impossible to predict the effect on the pressure gradient without knowing the original pressure gradient.

19. Which vessels anastomose to form the superior vena cava?

   a. right subclavian and left subclavian veins
   b. right subclavian and left innominate veins
   c. right innominate and left subclavian veins
   d. right innominate, right subclavian, and left brachiocephalic veins
   e. right innominate and left innominate veins

20. Which layer of an arterial or venous wall is composed entirely of endothelial tissue?

  a. tunica adventitia
  b. tunica media
  c. tunica intima
  d. None is composed of only one type of tissue.
  e. All layers are composed entirely of endothelial tissue.

21. In the normal anatomic position, which digit of the hand is the most lateral?

  a. digit #1
  b. digit #2
  c. digit #3
  d. digit #4
  e. digit #5

22. Which two factors determine kinetic energy?

  a. mass of the object and viscosity of fluid
  b. viscosity of fluid and velocity of the object
  c. mass of the object and velocity of the object
  d. velocity of the object and length of the segment
  e. potential energy and viscosity of fluid

23. What is the opening through which the internal maxillary artery passes as it exits onto the face?

  a. carotid canal
  b. supraorbital foramen
  c. infraorbital foramen
  d. infraorbital canal
  e. maxillary foramen

24. Which artery would you palpate slightly above and in front of the lateral malleolus?

  a. posterior tibial
  b. anterior tibial
  c. dorsalis pedis
  d. perineal
  e. peroneal

25. The name of the wall that divides the right and left ventricle is:

  a. ventricular wall
  b. intraventricular wall
  c. intraventricular septum
  d. interventricular septum
  e. interventricular valve

26. Which of the following statements is NOT true?

   a. Blood flows caudad in the abdominal aorta.
   b. Blood flows cephalad in the abdominal aorta.
   c. The abdominal aorta is inferior to the descending thoracic aorta.
   d. The abdominal aorta is superior to the common iliac arteries.
   e. The abdominal aorta is distal to the diaphragm.

27. Which artery is sometimes called the "artery of the leg"?

   a. common femoral artery
   b. profunda femoris
   c. superficial femoral
   d. popliteal
   e. deep femoral

28. Which two types of energy combine to determine fluid energy?

   a. potential and hydrostatic energy
   b. hydrostatic and kinetic energy
   c. kinetic and potential energy
   d. potential and mechanical energy
   e. kinetic and motion energy

29. What is the name of the arterial vessel that has only a tunica intima and a tunica media?

   a. artery
   b. arterial capillary
   c. venule
   d. arteriole
   e. There is none.

30. Which plane divides the body through the middle into top and bottom halves?

   a. coronal
   b. transverse
   c. sagittal
   d. median
   e. frontal

31. Which of these anatomic structures is found at the proximal border of the leg?

   a. inguinal ligament
   b. groin
   c. umbilicus
   d. ankle joint
   e. knee joint

32. Stroke volume is the:

a. volume of blood ejected from the heart each minute
b. volume of blood ejected from the left ventricle with each heartbeat
c. volume of blood ejected from the right ventricle with each heartbeat
d. volume of blood ejected from the left atrium with each heartbeat
e. volume of blood ejected from the right atrium with each heartbeat

33. The following vessel connects the right and left anterior cerebral arteries:

a. right and left posterior communicating arteries
b. middle cerebral artery
c. basilar artery
d. middle anterior artery
e. anterior communicating artery

34. Another name for the internal iliac artery is:

a. hypergastric artery
b. hypogastric artery
c. hyprogastric artery
d. internal gastric artery
e. internal pudendal artery

35. The muscle layer of the heart wall is called the:

a. epicardium
b. endocardium
c. adventitium
d. pericardium
e. myocardium

36. Which layer is sometimes called the muscle coat of an arterial wall?

a. tunica intima
b. tunica media
c. tunica adventitia
d. tunica myocardia
e. tunica pericardia

37. Which vessel layers are present in a venule?

a. tunica adventitia, tunica media, and tunica intima
b. tunica adventitia and tunica media
c. tunica adventitia and tunica intima
d. tunica media and tunica intima
e. tunica media and tunica adventitia

38. The digit commonly referred to as the ring finger is:

a. digit #1
b. digit #2
c. digit #3
d. digit #4
e. digit #5

39. Which two factors, alone or together, can cause energy losses in blood flow?

a. gravity or inertia
b. inertia or viscosity
c. viscosity or static filling pressure
d. static filling pressure or density
e. density or gravity

40. What is the other name for the innominate artery?

a. the internal iliac artery
b. the brachiocephalic artery
c. the hypogastric artery
d. the hypergastric artery
e. the hypocephalic artery

41. What happens to the heart rate with the stimulation of the pressoreceptor located in the carotid sinus?

a. There is no pressoreceptor in the carotid sinus, only a baroreceptor.
b. The heart rate can either increase or decrease, depending on the type of stimulation applied.
c. The heart rate is not affected in any way.
d. The heart rate increases.
e. The heart rate decreases.

42. What happens to the flow of venous blood out of the lower extremities in an upright body during expiration?

a. The flow rate decreases.
b. The flow rate increases.
c. Respiration has no effect on venous flow when a person is standing up.
d. It can either increase or decrease depending on leg muscle contraction.
e. The flow rate is never affected by expiration.

43. What are the three layers of the heart wall?

a. the pericardium, epicardium, and myocardium
b. the myocardium, pericardium, and endocardium
c. the endocardium, myocardium, and epicardium
d. the epicardium, endocardium, and myocardium
e. the pericardium, intracardium, and myocardium

44. What is defined as the pressure exerted by a fluid within a closed system?

a. gravitational potential energy
b. intravascular pressure
c. intervascular pressure
d. inertial pressure
e. hydrostatic pressure

45. What happens to the heart rate with stimulation of the pressoreceptor located in the aortic arch?

a. There is no pressoreceptor in the aortic arch, only a baroreceptor.
b. The heart rate can either increase or decrease, depending on the type of stimulation applied.
c. The heart rate is not affected in any way.
d. The heart rate increases.
e. The heart rate decreases.

46. Which of the following vessels is **NOT** a part of the external carotid artery family?

a. the internal maxillary artery
b. the superficial temporal artery
c. the occipital artery
d. the supraorbital artery
e. the infraorbital artery

47. In the normal anatomic position, which upper extremity digit is the most medial?

a. digit #1
b. digit #2
c. digit #3
d. digit #4
e. digit #5

48. What artery generally arises at the level of the carotid siphon?

a. the internal carotid artery
b. the ophthalmic artery
c. the middle meningeal artery
d. the supraorbital artery
e. the anterior cerebral artery

49. What is the first of the five major visceral branches of the abdominal aorta?

a. the celiac artery
b. the superior mesenteric artery
c. the hepatic artery
d. the inferior mesenteric artery
e. the splenic artery

50. What anatomic structure forms the distal border of the arm?

a. the fingers
b. the wrist
c. the elbow
d. the shoulder
e. the neck